COUNT OUT
CHOLESTEROL

COUNT OUT CHOLESTEROL

♥ ♥ ♥ ♥

Art Ulene, MD
Val Ulene, MD

Ulysses Press

1994

Published by: Ulysses Press
P.O. Box 3440
Berkeley, CA 94703-3440

Library of Congress Catalog Card Number 93-61557

ISBN 0-915233-96-7

First published in hardcover by Alfred A. Knopf, Inc. in 1989

Printed in the USA by The George Banta Company

10 9 8 7 6 5 4 3 2 1

Cover Design: Bonnie Smetts
Background photography: James Meyer/Image Bank
Ulene portrait: David Quinney
Color Separation: Re:Image

The weight charts on pages 73 and 74 are used courtesy of the Metropolitan Life Insurance Company.

The recipes in the book are © 1989 by The Hearst Corporation, and are reprinted with the permission of *Good Housekeeping* magazine.

Distributed in the United States by Publishers Group West, in Canada by Raincoast Books, and in Great Britain and Europe by World Leisure Marketing.

C O N T E N T S

♥ ♥ ♥ ♥

LIST OF CHARTS

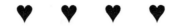

ACKNOWLEDGMENTS

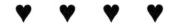

We gratefully acknowledge the contributions of: Richard Trubo, our primary writer, who worked tirelessly under pressure. His concern for accuracy and his attention to detail added immeasurably to this book.

To Toinette Lippe, our editor, for her insightful comments and her extraordinary patience.

Carol Wapner, RD, who created the recipes provided by the Good Housekeeping Institute, and to the Institute for sharing them with us.

James Anderson, MD, who kindly shared his research findings and gave generously of his time when we had questions, and to his associate, Libby Whitis-Clark, RD, who did the same.

Julie Zuckerman, whose meticulous research helped turn the "SF concept" into a workable system.

Jamie McDowell, who handled every administrative detail related to this book with skill and efficiency.

Neal Stone, MD, who reviewed the manuscript, enhancing it with his knowledge and expertise.

INTRODUCTION

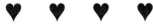

Just thirty years have passed since the modern battle against heart disease began in earnest. In that relatively short period of time, the mortality rate due to cardiovascular disease has fallen more than 40 percent. From 1980 to 1990, the death rate from heart attacks plummeted nearly 33 percent. The credit for these extraordinary results must be shared: by researchers who advanced our knowledge about heart disease and developed new methods for diagnosing and treating it; by practicing physicians who skillfully applied new knowledge and techniques in the care of their patients; and by people like you, for adopting healthier lifestyles that reduce the risk of coronary heart disease. Average blood cholesterol levels are declining, and we are clearly on the right track.

Nevertheless, more than 50 percent of all American adults still have blood cholesterol levels that are higher than the desirable range. Nearly half of this group have values over 240 mg/dl*, a level that more than doubles their risk of coronary heart disease. More than two of every five Americans still die of cardiovascular disease, with heart and blood disorders claiming 930,000 lives each year. A recent study by the U.S. Centers for Disease Control found that fewer than one-third of people who need a physician's treatment for high blood cholesterol levels are getting it.

It is you and the people like you who will determine how successful the campaign against heart disease will be in the years ahead. By applying the knowledge that has already been gained, you may be able to significantly reduce your own risk of coronary heart disease and reduce its impact on your health. If your blood cholesterol is high, and you are successful at lowering it, you may actually be able to *prevent* a heart attack.

For some people, the simple dietary changes described in this book will be all that is necessary to reduce blood cholesterol levels to a desirable range. For some, medical therapy may be necessary in addition. One way or another, using the methods described in this book, almost all people with high blood cholesterol can reduce their risk of coronary heart disease significantly—by as much as two percent for a one percent reduction in the blood cholesterol level.

If you have high blood cholesterol, we urge you to try to lower it now. Don't wait for the symptoms of coronary heart disease to appear before taking the steps that are necessary to bring your cholesterol level down into the healthy range. The earlier you start, the less likely you will be to ever experience those symptoms. At the very least, you may be able to delay the onset of heart disease, postponing it until much later in life, and thus giving you a higher quality of life for many more years. If you are reading this book because you already have symptoms of heart disease, or you have suffered a heart attack, don't be dismayed. There is now evidence that lowering cholesterol levels can halt the progress of atherosclerosis in many people—even reverse it in some. When that happens, your chances of having a heart attack will decline as well.

We urge you to join us in a program that can not only reduce your personal risk of heart disease, but enhance the quality of your life.

Arthur Ulene, MD
Val Ulene, MD

* Blood cholesterol levels are measured in milligrams per deciliter (e.g., 210 mg/dl); however, it is customary when talking about cholesterol to use only the number itself. For ease of reading, only the number will appear through most of this book.

PART 1

♥ ♥ ♥ ♥

GETTING READY TO COUNT

1

♥　♥　♥　♥

A SENSIBLE APPROACH

"My total cholesterol is 210. The magazine I read says that's very high. My doctor says I shouldn't worry. Who's right?"

"I'm trying to follow my doctor's diet for controlling cholesterol, but my friends laugh at the way I eat now. They say the cholesterol problem is overblown."

"I had my cholesterol measured at a shopping mall three times in the same day, and the numbers were all different. A report I saw on TV said that these tests aren't accurate, but the group that did my screening tests stands by the results."

"It says on the box that the crackers are made with 100 percent vegetable oil and they contain no cholesterol, but the dietician says I shouldn't eat them. Why?"

"I'd like to keep my cholesterol down, but I'm not willing to eat three oat bran muffins a day for the rest of my life. Are there any other foods that work just as well?"

These comments and questions are typical of the ones people are asking today. Unfortunately, many of the answers they are getting are either wrong, or confusing—or both.

The lady who asked if she should worry about her cholesterol of 210 was 88 years old, the perfect weight for her size, and the picture of health. A cholesterol level of 210 was probably the last thing she should have been worrying about that day.

The man who had his cholesterol screened three times in one day got the following results: 170, 164, and 176. Even though the numbers differ, they all lead to the same conclusion about his health, and they all fall within the acceptable accuracy range for blood cholesterol testing (a 5 percent error in either direction is considered acceptable).

The question about bran muffins is one that almost any of us might ask. Not everyone loves bran muffins. Even if you do like them, it is possible to get too much of a good thing. Fortunately, there are other foods you can eat that have the same cholesterol-lowering effect as oat bran.

Why are people still so confused about cholesterol? Why is there so much controversy? Don't we know everything about the subject yet? Are commercial interests deliberately clouding the issues? Are the "experts" coming up with too many simple answers for a complex problem? The last suggestion is probably closest to the mark. The fact is, there is no single approach that all of us can use to deal with the problem of high blood cholesterol, because we are all different. We are different biologically, we are different psychologically, and we choose to lead different lifestyles. Our approach to cholesterol must vary to accommodate those differences.

Some of us were born lucky—we inherited "good" genes, and our blood cholesterol levels stay low no matter what we eat. Others were born unlucky—we inherited a tendency toward very high blood cholesterol, so no matter how carefully we eat, it isn't enough to keep our cholesterol levels down in the desirable range. Most of us are in the middle—our genetic makeup allows our cholesterol levels to move up and down according to how we eat. And since most of us don't eat as well as we should, both our cholesterol levels and our risk of heart disease are higher than they should be.

Because we are all different, it doesn't make sense to give everyone the same advice, but that is happening all too often. Health food faddists tell us we should lower blood cholesterol levels with high (sometimes toxic) doses of vitamins. Television talk show guests advise us to eat three oat bran muffins a day for the rest of our lives. And self-styled experts tell us (incorrectly) that it doesn't matter what we eat as long as we take one of the modern cholesterol-lowering drugs.

If your blood cholesterol level is high, you don't want that kind of advice. You need to know what's causing *your* cholesterol to be high, and you need advice that will help you correct the underlying problem instead of just treating the symptom.

This book is designed to help you do just that. In it, you'll learn the different reasons why people develop high blood cholesterol, and you'll discover what steps can be taken to correct each problem. By concentrating on two dietary factors—saturated fat and soluble fiber—you'll discover ways to lower your cholesterol level without a rigid diet, without boring foods, and without great sacrifice. You'll learn about other lifestyle changes that can not only reduce your risk of developing coronary heart disease but also improve the way you feel. For many people, these dietary and lifestyle measures will be all that is necessary to bring their cholesterol levels down into the desirable range; but if you are one of those who needs more intensive treatment to reduce their cholesterol level to a healthier level, you'll learn what medical therapies are available to help you.

HOW IS *COUNT OUT CHOLESTEROL* DIFFERENT?

If you are interested in the subject of cholesterol—especially if you have a problem with it yourself—you are probably well aware of the many solutions that have been suggested for high blood cholesterol. Government agencies advise you to cut your fat intake to less than 30 percent of your total calories. One best-selling author tells you that oat bran can save your life, while another claims that fish oils are the key to success. The health food stores sell niacin for lowering cholesterol, while the pharmaceutical companies offer prescription medications. Who's right?

To some extent, they all are. Cutting the amount of fat you eat each day may reduce your blood cholesterol level 5–15 percent, but you shouldn't stop there. Fish, rich in omega-3 fatty acids, are another potent weapon you can use. Oat bran may help you lower your cholesterol, too, but it is not the only source of fiber that will accomplish this. By reducing the amount of cholesterol your liver makes, niacin may lower your blood cholesterol level; but it takes high doses of niacin to do this, and if its use is not monitored, closely, there may be toxic side effects. So, if you need a drug to bring your cholesterol to a desirable range, one of several available prescription drugs—or niacin—may be the best choice in your particular case. None of them should be taken, however, without a physician's supervision.

For some people, any one of these solutions may be all that is needed to get their cholesterol levels down as low as they should be. But most people can benefit from combining two of these steps (such as reducing fat *and* increasing soluble fiber in the diet), and some people may need to try *all* of them before finding the right combination. We are not alike, so it's important to know about every option available if you have high blood cholesterol.

That's what you'll find in *Count Out Cholesterol*. You'll not only learn how to reduce dietary fats, but how to specifically target the fats that cause most of the trouble—saturated fats. You will find out how a dietary substance called soluble fiber can decrease your cholesterol level even more—much more. And you will discover many different sources of soluble fiber, so your diet can continue to be varied and enjoyable. For many people, these dietary alterations will be all that's necessary to lower their blood cholesterol level into the desirable range. If these measures still aren't enough to get your cholesterol where it ought to be, your doctor will work with you to find the best medical therapy available.

This program cannot promise that your cholesterol level will drop by a specific amount, because each individual is different, and each responds differently to these cholesterol-lowering measures. We *can* assure you that you'll enjoy following the plan. This book contains no rigid menus you must follow, no special recipes you must prepare, and no specific foods you must eat. Instead, it is filled with facts and principles that you can use every day to design your own menus and to adapt your own recipes. If you have a family, everyone can participate with you and enjoy the benefits of this healthy lifestyle.

This approach has been chosen because most people benefit more from learning and using these general principles than from being forced to follow a rigid program. This plan allows you much greater flexibility in your busy schedule and much more freedom to lead your normal lifestyle. It's also a program you can follow for the rest of your life.

HOW FAST CAN YOU GET YOUR CHOLESTEROL DOWN?

According to the National Cholesterol Education Program (which is coordinated by the National Heart, Lung, and Blood Institute), the average person on a cholesterol-lowering diet will decrease his cholesterol level gradually, reaching the lowest achievable point over a period of about six months.

However, research shows that this level can be reached by some individuals much more quickly. Decreasing dietary fat alone has been shown to reduce blood cholesterol levels by as much as 10 percent in just seven days. When such a diet is continued, the cholesterol levels continue to fall, reaching a total drop of 12.5 percent at four weeks and 15 percent after two months. Though these rapid changes do not happen with

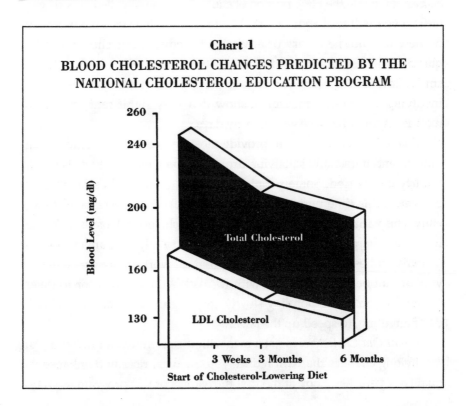

Chart 1
BLOOD CHOLESTEROL CHANGES PREDICTED BY THE NATIONAL CHOLESTEROL EDUCATION PROGRAM

everyone, they are achievable by many people, and may produce larger declines in individuals with very high cholesterol levels.

People who are overweight may also enjoy certain advantages when it comes to lowering cholesterol. If you are obese, you're more likely to have a high cholesterol level than if you are thin. However, by losing weight, you've got a better chance of getting your cholesterol level down. In fact, overweight individuals have the potential to cut their cholesterol more significantly and rapidly than people of average weight, just by losing ten, twenty, or more pounds.

Perhaps the most dramatic example of the speed and extent to which cholesterol levels can be lowered was provided by a bold group of Finnish researchers in 1984. They studied thirteen middle-aged women and ten men who walked 215 miles in seven days, during which time they drank water, mineral drinks, and fruit juices, but ate no food (we definitely do not recommend this approach for reducing cholesterol). By the end of seven days, their average total blood cholesterol level had fallen by almost 30 percent, while the HDL portion of cholesterol (the so-called "good" cholesterol you will read about shortly) had risen. While from a medical point of view it is not necessary or advisable to reduce your cholesterol that quickly (and not worth the risks and extraordinary effort involved), this study shows that rapid reduction is certainly possible. Many other studies, involving less drastic measures, show that very significant cholesterol reductions can take place within thirty days.

Count Out Cholesterol will provide most people with a medically significant and personally satisfying drop in blood cholesterol levels within a thirty-day period. Some people may lower their level as much as 30 percent in this time period, but to repeat, everyone will respond differently. This variation in the rate and amount of cholesterol loss is a uniquely human characteristic, and is why we need to rely on human (not just animal) studies to guide us. So if the program works more gradually for you, do not become impatient with it. Work with your doctor to determine why you are responding slowly and to learn what else you should do, if anything, to speed up the pace.

Count Out Cholesterol is not a race with the calendar, but rather a plan for lifelong changes that will reduce your medical risks and enhance the quality of your life. Look at the first thirty days of this program as an opportunity to demonstrate how your body reacts to the healthful changes you are making, and enjoy the fact that you can make these alterations safely and without any real sacrifices.

This book is one that you can pick up again and again. Make some positive changes now, and then in the weeks and months ahead, make some others. If you get off to a slow start, perhaps achieving only limited declines in your cholesterol, keep in mind that the process will get easier. As you acquire knowledge about the importance of bringing your cholesterol under control, that knowledge will become powerful. It will help you learn and master the skills necessary for reducing your cholesterol.

2

♥ ♥ ♥ ♥

CHOLESTEROL DOES COUNT

The controversy is over. For many years, scientists argued about the role that the fatty substance called cholesterol plays in the development of heart disease. Everyone agreed that cholesterol could be found blocking the blood vessels that supply oxygen to the heart muscle, and it was common knowledge that people with high blood cholesterol levels had more heart attacks than those with low levels. However, the arguments were loud and long about what role dietary cholesterol played in causing the trouble, and what effect dietary changes could have in preventing it.

For almost thirty years, researchers have been trying to settle these issues with carefully controlled scientific studies. Their suspicions about cholesterol's role were aroused by the observation that the incidence of coronary heart disease varied from country to country in relation to the amount of fat in the general diet. In countries where high fat diets were common, the rate of heart disease was high. Where the diet was very low in fat, so, too, was the incidence of heart disease.

Chart 2

CHOLESTEROL LEVELS IN DIFFERENT COUNTRIES

East Finland	265
West Finland	253
Former Soviet Union	236
Holland	230
Crete, Greece	206
Montegiorgio, Italy	198
Corfu, Greece	198
Dalmatia, Croatia	186
Tanushimaru, Japan	171
Ushibuka, Japan	141

These numbers represent the 50th percentile for blood cholesterol levels in each country (the 50th percentile is the level below or above which 50 percent of the population fell) For example, 50 percent of the men in East Finland had cholesterol levels below 265, while half had levels above that figure By contrast, the 50th percentile cholesterol level for men in Ushibuka, Japan, was 141.

The importance of blood cholesterol was suggested by further research which showed that average blood cholesterol levels also varied greatly from country to country, moving up or down in relation to the amount of fat in each country's diet and rate of heart disease. Chart 2 shows how much the average blood cholesterol level of men aged 40 to 59 varied, in one study, from country to country, and even from region to region within the same country.

No matter what country was studied, one fact quickly became clear: The men* with the highest cholesterol levels had much higher rates of heart attacks than those with low cholesterol levels. In one ten-year study, researchers followed more than 10,000 men who were believed to be free of heart disease and whose cholesterol levels were known. Chart 3 reveals the percentage of men at each cholesterol level who died of cardiovascular disease during this ten-year period. As you can see, the frequency of heart-disease deaths increased dramatically as cholesterol levels rose—from less than a 1 percent death rate (cholesterol level: 160-179) to more than a 9 percent rate (cholesterol level: greater than 300).

---

* To date, most cholesterol studies have focused primarily on men, since they account for most cases of heart disease.

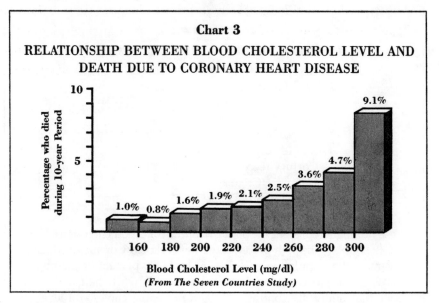

Chart 3

RELATIONSHIP BETWEEN BLOOD CHOLESTEROL LEVEL AND DEATH DUE TO CORONARY HEART DISEASE

Blood Cholesterol Level (mg/dl)
(From The Seven Countries Study)

The message is clear: The likelihood that a person will develop coronary heart disease (narrowing down and blockage of the arteries that supply blood to the heart muscle) is directly related to the amount of cholesterol he or she has in the blood. The higher the level of blood cholesterol, the greater the risk of coronary heart disease. Cholesterol *does* count.

It was once thought that the amount of cholesterol in your blood had to rise above a certain level (the so-called "risk threshold") before your risk of heart disease started to go up. As recently as the late 1970s, many scientists and physicians insisted that your blood cholesterol level was not abnormal until it exceeded 300, because they believed that the risk of heart disease was not increased until that level was reached.

Newer studies show that the risk of a heart attack actually begins to rise as the total blood cholesterol level passes 140 to 150, and continues to increase as the cholesterol level goes up. The Framingham Heart Study, probably the best-known study of heart disease in the United States, examined this issue in depth. Researchers have kept constant track of the health of nearly the entire population of Framingham, Massachusetts, since 1948. They found that the risk of a heart attack begins to rise gradually around 150 and then increases more steeply after the level exceeds 200. Their study reveals that an individual whose total blood cholesterol level is 300 has about four times the risk of coronary heart disease than a person whose level is 200. Though the risk is quite small below 150, Framingham's researchers concluded that *no* cholesterol level will guarantee that an individual is free of all risk of developing coronary heart disease. Those findings have been confirmed in other studies, one of which is graphically represented in Chart 4.

This large study, humorously referred to as MR. FIT (the initials stand for Multiple Risk Factor Intervention Trial), reached similar conclusions. Its investigators evaluated over 360,000 men from eighteen U.S. cities. In 1986, they reported that blood cholesterol levels which many

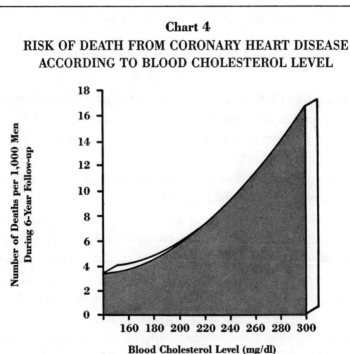

Chart 4

RISK OF DEATH FROM CORONARY HEART DISEASE ACCORDING TO BLOOD CHOLESTEROL LEVEL

This chart is based on a study of 361,662 men aged 35 to 57 who were followed for an average of about six years. The figures on the left represent the number of men per thousand who died from coronary heart disease during the six-year period. For example, among men whose cholesterol levels were 180, four per thousand died. Approximately seven per thousand died among men whose cholesterol levels were 220. Notice that the risk of dying from a heart attack increases continuously as the blood cholesterol level rises. The pace at which the risk increases begins to accelerate after the cholesterol level passes 200.

physicians once considered safe are actually associated with an increased risk of death from coronary heart disease. For example, men with cholesterol levels between 203 and 220 mg/dl had a 73 percent higher coronary death rate than men with values of 181 or under. Even men with levels between 182 and 202 had a 29 percent greater chance of dying from coronary heart disease than those with levels of 181 or below.

At the time these studies were going on, the average blood cholesterol level for middle-aged American males was around 220, and most men in the U.S. were being told that anything between 180 and 280 was "normal." In a statistical sense, that may have been true, but it certainly wouldn't have been normal in other parts of the world, where diets were lower in fat. For example, in the Orient, where the incidence of heart attacks was low, the average cholesterol level of a middle-aged man was closer to 160.

Another group of investigators set out to examine the effect lowering blood cholesterol had on the risk of heart attack. The Lipid Research Clinics Coronary Primary Prevention Trial involved 3,806 middle-aged men (ages 35 to 59) with high blood cholesterol levels (averaging about 292). In this study, half of the subjects were given a cholesterol-lowering drug called cholestyramine; others received a placebo (an inactive pill). Both groups also went on a low-fat diet. After seven to ten years of follow-up, the results were dramatic: The men receiving both drug and dietary therapy experienced an 8.5 percent greater reduction in blood cholesterol than the diet-only group, and that translated into a 19 percent decline in heart attacks. With each incremental decrease in cholesterol, there was an additional reduction in the risk of a heart attack. This was the first such study to demonstrate clearly that lowering blood cholesterol levels would actually reduce the incidence of heart attacks.

This same study also found improvements in other areas: The treated group had 20 percent fewer new cases of angina (chest pain), 21 percent fewer coronary bypass surgeries, and 25 percent fewer abnormalities on exercise electrocardiograms. Thus, as cholesterol levels dropped, so did heart disease and all its associated problems. Based on their results, researchers concluded that if your blood cholesterol level is high, for each 1 percent you can lower it, you can reduce your chances of coronary heart disease by about 2 percent. That would mean that lowering your cholesterol 15 percent—from 250 to 212, for example—could make your risk of a heart attack fall by as much as 30 percent!

That is apparently the case, but this formula is applicable only up to a point. If you were able to reduce your cholesterol level by 50 percent (perhaps from 320 to 160), you could not expect your risk of coronary heart disease to fall 100 percent—or literally to zero. No matter how well you do in reducing your cholesterol, there's no guarantee that you'll never experience a heart attack. Even so, this two-to-one guideline is an indication of just how significant each incremental decline in your total cholesterol level can be

As researchers began to study cholesterol in greater and greater depth, they discovered the rather astonishing fact that some cholesterol, found in a particle in the blood known as "high density lipoprotein," and referred to as "HDL cholesterol could actually have the opposite effect on the incidence of heart attacks. It appeared to prevent them. Some of the most persuasive evidence for this comes from the Framingham Heart Study. In 1986, for instance, investigators there reported on the relationship between HDL cholesterol and heart disease in men and women age forty-nine or over. Whether an individual's total cholesterol was high or low, the risk of heart disease was cut as HDL levels rose. Those people who had high HDL concentrations (at the 80th percentile) had half the risk of heart disease as those with low concentrations (at the 20th percentile).

A 1987 scientific report added weight to the theory that the risk of heart attacks could be reduced by measures that made HDL cholesterol levels go up. Researchers with the Helsinki Heart Study published their findings involving more than 4,000 middle-aged men with elevated cholesterol levels (an average of 270). These individuals received either the cholesterol-lowering drug gemfibrozil or a placebo for five years. Compared to the placebo group, the individuals taking gemfibrozil experienced an average decrease of eight percent in their total cholesterol level. Based on the two-to-one formula cited above, you would expect this 8 percent drop in cholesterol to result in a 16 percent decline in heart attacks. But, in fact, the results were much more impressive. The incidence of coronary heart disease was 34 percent lower in the drug group. At the same time, the death rate from coronary heart disease was 26 percent lower.

Why were these declines in heart attacks so large? Researchers believe that increases in HDL (of about 10 percent) and/or decreases in blood triglycerides (a form of fat) in these men probably deserve the credit. In other words, even these moderate improvements in HDL cholesterol appeared to play an important role in slashing heart attack risks. Ironically, despite the positive findings in both the Helsinki Heart Study and the Lipid Research Clinics Coronary Primary Prevention Trials, these studies were criticized because they did not show a decline in *total* mortality. However, neither study had numbers large enough to demonstrate decreases in total mortality, even if one existed, and in fact, they had never been designed to do so. Nevertheless, keep in mind that both *did* show declines in heart attacks and in deaths from coronary heart disease, which are powerful reasons to bring your cholesterol levels under control.

Chart 5

ABOUT TRIGLYCERIDES

Triglycerides are a type of fatty substance that your doctor may talk about as you work together on your cholesterol-lowering program. Blood triglyceride levels tend to be elevated in people who have high cholesterol levels, in people with diabetes or chronic kidney disease, and in those who are obese.

The relationship between triglycerides and coronary heart disease is still controversial. Although some studies suggest that high blood triglyceride levels might increase the risk of coronary heart disease, other research fails to substantiate this association. However, there does appear to be a link between high triglycerides, low HDL levels, and forms of LDL that are particularly prone to form plaques on arterial walls.

If your blood triglyceride level is markedly elevated, your physician may recommend therapy designed to lower it. This can be accomplished by dietary change, exercise, and weight loss in most people. The use of medication to lower triglycerides while improving HDL and LDL readings may be necessary in some cases. The issue of triglycerides is complicated, however, because levels can become so variable, changing as much as 100 points from one measurement to the next. Stress, diet, and physical activity can greatly influence a particular triglyceride reading. For example, if an individual has not fasted for at least 12 hours before testing, the measurement may not be reliable.

Even before the Helsinki study, some cholesterol experts believed that HDL was a so-called "independent risk factor" for heart disease. In other words, they said, if you can increase your HDL cholesterol levels, that in itself will decrease your chances of having a heart attack, no matter what happens to your overall total cholesterol levels.

As total cholesterol declines and HDL rises, why does the rate of heart attacks fall? Researchers have documented that at the same time, real changes are taking place in the coronary arteries. Angiograms (special x-rays of the arteries) have confirmed that reducing the cholesterol level will, in some people, slow down or even reverse the buildup of fatty deposits in the coronary arteries that can ultimately lead to a heart attack.

One of the first studies that used angiograms to demonstrate this was the National Heart, Lung, and Blood Institute (NHLBI) Type II Coronary Intervention Study, published in 1984. It divided patients with high cholesterol levels into two groups—one received cholestyramine (the cholesterol-lowering drug) plus a special diet, while the other was placed on a placebo and the same diet. When they joined the study, all of the patients had narrowing of their coronary arteries, confirmed by angiograms. Five years after this investigation began, repeat angiograms and other tests were conducted, with impressive results. Not only had cholesterol levels dropped by 17 percent in the patients receiving the drug and diet regimen, but the narrowing of their arteries had progressed much less than among the placebo group. Among those with the most serious lesions, one-third of the placebo patients experienced a worsening of their atherosclerosis—hardening of the arteries—compared to only 12 percent in the drug group.

Even more startling were the results of a study published in 1987, which revealed that it may be possible to *reverse* atherosclerotic blockage of the arteries. Just ten years earlier, most scientists would have scoffed at the suggestion that hardening of the arteries due to cholesterol deposits could be reversed, but Dr. David Blankenhorn and his colleagues at the University of Southern California decided to test this notion. They recruited a group of 162 men (ages 40 to 59) who had previously undergone coronary bypass surgery. Angiograms were performed to confirm that these men had blockage in their arteries, and the researchers measured the exact size of the openings that remained in the blood vessels. Half of the subjects were placed on a strict low-fat, low-cholesterol diet and cho-lesterol-lowering drugs (colestipol and niacin). The other half were given a less restricted low-fat diet and a placebo instead of drugs.

The results: The drug-treated men experienced an average 26 percent drop in their total blood cholesterol (from 246 to 180), compared to 4 per-cent in the other group. Perhaps even more significantly, repeat angio-grams taken after the two-year study revealed that blockages in the coronary arteries had actually *regressed* in 16 percent of the men on the strict diet and drug regimen. In another 45 percent, the lesions were unchanged, indicating that the deterioration process had been halted. Even in the men receiving the low-fat diet without drugs, 37 percent had unchanged lesions, and about 2 percent showed a regression. In this placebo group, the lower the fat content in the diet, the better. While those volunteers who ate a higher-fat diet (34 percent of calories from fat) tend-ed to develop new fatty deposits, those consuming a lower-fat diet (28 percent of calories from fat) tended to have no progression of the block-ages in their arteries. The proof was there: Atherosclerosis *could* be halted and, in some cases, reversed.

Incidentally, while reading the studies cited above, you may have noticed that in most cases, cholesterol-lowering drugs were used to achieve the major improvements in cholesterol levels. In most of these large studies, the participants were individuals with very high choles-terol levels, and researchers gave drugs to some of them as one means of dealing with their condition. That raises the question—since the empha-sis of this book is upon *non*-drug approaches to lowering cholesterol—can you expect the same changes in your heart-attack risk by following the program described in this book without drugs?

Actually, there is every reason to believe that the same positive changes can be achieved without medications. Dr. Dean Ornish at the University of California at San Francisco School of Medicine has con-ducted some of the most impressive research demonstrating that lifestyle changes alone can reverse heart disease. In one study, a group of Dr. Ornish's heart disease patients made significant changes in their diet and lifestyle, including adopting a very low-fat vegetarian diet, in which only 10 percent of calories came from fat. They ate no animal products except for egg whites and a cup of skim milk or yogurt per day. They also participated in a stress reduction program and moderate exercise, and they stopped smoking. Another group of patients—the "control" group—were not instructed to make changes in their lifestyle, and maintained a diet in which they consumed about 30 percent of their calories from dietary fat.

A year later, angiograms showed that 82 percent of the treatment group experienced changes toward reversal of the blockages in their coronary arteries, along with a decline in total cholesterol of 24 percent. By comparison, 53 percent of those in the control group showed progression, or worsening, of their disease.

Dr. Ornish's diet, however, was extremely restrictive. Most people would have difficulty adhering to a diet composed of only 10 percent fat, and thus the program has been criticized by some people (not us), as impractical. But that isn't the case with the lifestyle plan utilized in the STARS (St. Thomas Atherosclerosis Regression Study) trial. Ninety men with coronary heart disease were divided into three groups: those adopting a low-fat diet; those consuming the same diet, while also taking cholesterol-lowering drugs (cholestyramine); and those receiving "usual" care without any dietary changes or medication. The low-fat diet was quite similar to the one you will find in this book. Total fat intake was 27 percent of calories and saturated fat intake was 8 to 10 percent of calories. There were also limitations on dietary cholesterol, and increases in fiber consumption.

The research team, headed by Dr. D. F. Watts and Dr. B. Lewis at St. Thomas' Hospital in London, found that after more than three years, the low-fat diet alone had not only slowed progression of coronary disease, but in some patients, had produced regression of their arterial blockages. At the same time, they had fewer heart attacks, strokes, and heart bypass surgeries than the control group. The group adopting dietary changes plus drug therapy was even more effective, producing more regression and similar improvements in heart attacks and other cardiac events.

Other studies will be described throughout this book showing that non-drug approaches (from dietary changes to exercise) *can* improve your cholesterol level. Many experts believe that a cholesterol level lowered this way should have the same likelihood of stopping or reversing atherosclerosis in the coronary arteries as a cholesterol level lowered by drugs.

Until all the results are in, you have nothing to lose (except weight)—and probably a lot to gain—by following the entire program in this book, including diet and exercise. If you conscientiously adhere to these recommendations, your total cholesterol should decline. As it does, there is an excellent chance that your risk of heart disease will fall as well.

In 1987, when the National Cholesterol Education Program panel of experts met to examine the latest evidence on the subject, their report included an ominous message: *One-quarter of all American adults have cholesterol levels above 240, a level that greatly increases their risk.* This report—and a second report issued in 1993—also contained some good news: There are many ways to lower those cholesterol levels and reduce the risk. If you are one of the people with high blood cholesterol, don't wait for the symptoms of heart disease to appear before you make the corrective changes. The earlier you start, the less likely you will be to ever experience those symptoms.

If you lower your cholesterol, you may be able to save your life. It's as simple and significant as that.

3

♥ ♥ ♥ ♥

WHAT DETERMINES YOUR CHOLESTEROL LEVEL?

Cholesterol is a waxy, odorless substance that is found in foods of animal origin, including beef, poultry, fish, cheese, eggs, and dairy products. In general, the more cholesterol you put into your body by eating such foods, the higher your blood cholesterol concentration will be. But dietary cholesterol is not the only determinant of your blood cholesterol level. The amount of fat (especially saturated fat) you eat, and the amount of cholesterol your liver manufactures on its own, also play important roles.

The body requires some cholesterol for good health. Cholesterol is used to build the walls of cells throughout your body and to manufacture other essential substances, like hormones and vitamin D; in very young children, cholesterol plays an important role in the development of the brain. So it's important to have some cholesterol circulating throughout the bloodstream at all times. It is only when the amount of cholesterol in the blood becomes too high that health hazards begin to appear.

Pure cholesterol can't mix with or dissolve in solutions like water and blood, so it is combined in your liver with other substances (fats and proteins) to form particles that are capable of moving through the bloodstream. These particles, called lipoproteins, carry cholesterol from the liver to all parts of the body where it is needed, and then bring it back again for removal from the body. There are several different types of lipoproteins, including:

Very low density lipoproteins (VLDLs, or VLDL cholesterol)
Low density lipoproteins (LDLs, or LDL cholesterol)
High density lipoproteins (HDLs, or HDL cholesterol)

Each of these cholesterol forms can be measured separately in your blood. Together they make up your "total blood cholesterol" or "total cholesterol."

Very Low Density Lipoproteins (VLDLs)

The liver combines cholesterol, proteins, and fats (including triglycerides, which are blood fats) to form very low density lipoproteins, or VLDLs. These particles derive their name from the relatively low weight or density of their protein. As these VLDLs travel throughout the body, most of the triglycerides are removed, either for energy or to be stored as fat. In the process, the VLDLs are eventually converted to LDLs, which are described below.

Low Density Lipoproteins (LDLs)

Once triglycerides are removed from the VLDLs, the smaller particles that remain contain mostly cholesterol and protein. These particles are called low density lipoproteins, or LDLs. Many of these LDLs are removed from the bloodstream by cells throughout the body; in the cells, they are broken down into their original elements and used for essential bodily functions. However, this process does not always progress smoothly. Some people's systems remove LDLs more slowly than others, and this causes the level of LDLs (and thus cholesterol) to build up in their blood. (This tendency to remove LDLs and cholesterol quickly or slowly is inherited.)

If the blood levels of LDL cholesterol become too high, there is a tendency for the cholesterol and other fatty substances to deposit in the walls of arteries. This process, known as atherosclerosis, gradually narrows the arteries and chokes off the flow of blood through them. This is the reason why LDLs have gained the nickname "bad" cholesterol—they are the real culprit in the development of coronary heart disease that is due to high blood cholesterol. In this book, when we talk about getting your blood cholesterol level down, we are really concerned about decreasing the LDL portion of it.

In most people, about 60–70 percent of all the cholesterol in the blood is in the form of LDLs, so if your LDL cholesterol level is very high, your total blood cholesterol level is likely to be high, too. Also, if your LDL level goes up or down significantly, your total blood cholesterol level will tend to rise or fall significantly. That is why the less expensive measurement of "total cholesterol" is often used to screen people for cholesterol problems and to monitor people who are trying to lower their levels.

High Density Lipoproteins (HDLs)

Though HDLs also contain some cholesterol combined with proteins and fats, these particles have a very different effect within the body. HDLs act as scavengers or "vacuum cleaners" within the bloodstream, attracting cholesterol and carrying it *back* to the liver, where it is either reprocessed into new VLDL particles, or broken down into substances called bile acids and removed from the body. This helps to *reduce* the amount of cholesterol that is present in the blood and available to damage arteries. For that reason, HDL cholesterol has been nicknamed "good cholesterol." As we pointed out in Chapter Two, the higher your HDL cholesterol level, the less risk you will generally have of developing coronary heart disease.

WHAT DETERMINES YOUR
TOTAL CHOLESTEROL LEVEL?

Everyone, then, has some cholesterol in the bloodstream—that's a desirable situation. What we're concerned about is *excess* cholesterol—a condition that can be caused by several different factors. Although some of these causes are beyond your control, most are quite manageable, providing you with several different ways you can influence your own cholesterol level. Let's look now at the factors that determine what your blood cholesterol level will be.

Intrinsic Factors

Intrinsic factors are those that are "built into" your body makeup and therefore tend to be out of your direct control. They include heredity, age, and sex. Heredity plays perhaps the most important role, by determining how rapidly LDL cholesterol is removed from your bloodstream and how much new cholesterol is manufactured by your liver.

As pointed out earlier, even if there is no cholesterol in the foods you eat, your liver should produce as much cholesterol as your body needs for good health. However, some people inherit a tendency to overproduce cholesterol. Their livers produce *much* more than their bodies could ever utilize. These individuals may have total cholesterol readings as high as 400, 500, or even more—levels that are very dangerously elevated. Such high levels predispose people to the development of atherosclerosis at a very young age and to the occurrence of heart attacks as early as their thirties and forties. In rare severe cases, heart attacks can even occur in childhood. This type of cholesterol problem runs in families, so if your mother or father had an extremely high cholesterol level, you may have inherited the tendency.

Another intrinsic factor that influences your blood cholesterol level is your age. As you grow older, your total blood cholesterol level will tend naturally to rise. As a result, a seventy-year-old man with a cholesterol count of 215 may not have nearly as much to worry about as a thirty-five-year-old man with the same reading.

Your sex is also an influence upon your susceptibility to heart disease. The male sex is much more at risk than females; particularly before menopause, women are less vulnerable to a heart attack. Studies show that women tend to have higher HDL ("good") cholesterol levels than men of the same age. However, this natural advantage of women can be overshadowed by other factors, such as the use of oral contraceptives or estrogens. Some types of birth control pills may raise the total cholesterol level slightly, while lowering the HDL cholesterol count—both undesirable consequences. The effect that oral contraceptives have on cholesterol can vary considerably, depending on the proportions of estrogen and progesterone in the pills (it may differ from one brand to another). If you are using birth control pills and you have high blood cholesterol, your doctor may want to measure your cholesterol level more frequently to monitor this potential effect.

Even though you can't change your heredity, your age, or your sex, you *can* compensate for any problems they cause by making a real effort to manage those factors that *are* subject to your control. Let's take a look at these influences.

Intake Factors

Intake factors are those related to the food you eat. They are extremely important for most people with cholesterol problems because they usually have a significant effect on the blood cholesterol level and because they can easily be controlled. The most important intake factors are saturated fats and dietary cholesterol—in that order.

Biochemists classify fats into three major categories—saturated, polyunsaturated, and monounsaturated—based on a certain characteristic of their chemical structure (namely, the number of hydrogen atoms they have). Although most foods (even some plant-derived foods) contain a combination of all three types of fats, one of them usually predominates. Thus, a food is considered "saturated" or "high in saturates" when it's composed primarily of saturated fatty acids (the carbon atoms in their molecular framework are "saturated" with hydrogen atoms, or incapable of absorbing any more of them). By contrast, a food composed mostly of polyunsaturated or monounsaturated fatty acids is called "polyunsaturated" or "monounsaturated" (the fat molecules have room for additional hydrogen atoms).

Saturated fats tend to harden at room temperature, and are found primarily in animal products, particularly fatty meats (beef, veal, lamb, pork, ham) and many dairy items (whole milk, cream, ice cream, cheese). For example, the marbleized fat you can see on beef is saturated. Some types of vegetable products—coconut oil, palm oil, palm kernel oil, and vegetable shortening—are also high in saturates. Because they are inexpensive and taste good, these highly saturated vegetable fats are frequently used in commercially baked goods and snack foods such as cookies and crackers.

The liver uses saturated fats to manufacture cholesterol. Therefore, excessive dietary intake of saturated fats can significantly raise the blood cholesterol, especially in people who have inherited a tendency toward high blood cholesterol. Guidelines issued by the National Cholesterol Education Program and widely supported by most experts recommend that your intake of saturated fats should be less than 10 percent of your total calorie intake (in Chapter Eight, you will learn how to determine that level quickly and easily). However, for people who have severe problems with high blood cholesterol, even that level may be too high.

Polyunsaturated fats, on the other hand, may actually lower your total blood cholesterol level. However, in doing so, large amounts of polyunsaturates also have a tendency to reduce your HDL ("good") cholesterol level, so it makes no sense to overdo your intake of this kind of fat. Several vegetable oils are rich in polyunsaturated fats, particularly corn, soybean, safflower, and sunflower seed oil. Also, certain fish oils, particularly the omega-3 fatty acids, are high in polyunsaturates.

The National Cholesterol Education Program guidelines recommend that your intake of polyunsaturated fats should not exceed 10 percent of your total calorie intake. This is especially good advice if you are trying to control your weight since these fats—as all other types—are very high in calories for their weight and volume.

Monounsaturated fats appear to reduce blood levels of LDL cholesterol without affecting HDL in any way. However, this positive impact upon LDL cholesterol is relatively modest. Monounsaturated fats are found in oils—especially olive and peanut oils—and are also prevalent in some margarines. The National Cholesterol Education Program guidelines recommend that your intake of monounsaturated fats be between 10 and 15 percent of your total calorie intake. Because the LDL-lowering effect of monosaturated fats is modest, and especially because the calorie content of these foods is very high, eating large quantities of monounsaturates is not a good strategy for lowering your LDL.

One other element could become an important factor in the cholesterol equation. Recent research into *trans fatty acids* suggests that they, too, might play a detrimental role in blood cholesterol levels. Trans fatty acids are fats that have been manipulated molecularly into new configurations in the laboratory, often as a way to harden liquid vegetable oils for use in foods like margarine and shortening. One recent study found that trans monounsaturated fatty acids raised LDL cholesterol levels, so that they behaved much like saturated fats; simultaneously, these same trans fatty acids reduced HDL cholesterol readings.

Much more research is still necessary, since some studies have not produced clear-cut conclusions about these trans fatty acids. But your dietary choices could become less matter-of-fact than they now appear. For now, however, from a cholesterol-lowering point of view, polyunsaturated and monounsaturated fats are much more desirable than saturated fats. As a general rule, the NCEP recommends that you maintain about equal amounts of each in your diet (with perhaps a little more emphasis upon monounsaturated rather than polyunsaturated fats). The NCEP guidelines also recommend that you keep your total fat intake at 30 percent or below of your daily calorie intake (in our opinion, the farther below, the better). The table on page 31 will guide you toward making rational choices.

Ironically, when people have been forced by circumstance to eat a healthier, lower-fat diet, their well-being has improved. In some parts of Europe during World War II, fatty foods simply weren't available. The result was a remarkable decline in coronary heart disease, despite the high stress of living in wartime.

A dramatic example of the effect of dietary fat and cholesterol on Coronary Heart Disease (CHD) has come from studies of Japanese men who have moved from their own country to the U.S. Japan has a relatively low rate of CHD, in large part due to a diet that stresses low saturated fat foods such as fish. However, when these emigrants moved from Japan to Hawaii or San Francisco—and adopted typical Western diets that were higher in total fat, saturated fat, and dietary cholesterol—their blood cholesterol levels rose, as did their CHD death rates. It was their diet, not genetics, that produced these undesirable changes in blood cholesterol and heart disease.

Excellent studies—dating back more than two decades—have also examined the relationship between blood cholesterol levels and saturated fats, and concluded that these fats have more of a detrimental impact upon cholesterol concentrations than any other nutritional factor, including dietary cholesterol.

In the Seven Countries Study, published in 1970, the diets and health status of fourteen population groups living in seven different nations were compared. Each of these groups was composed of at least 500 men, ranging in age from 40 to 59 years. By comparing the types of fats and other nutritional components in these men's diet, researchers found that 80 percent of the differences in blood cholesterol levels among the groups were due to variations in the amount of saturated fat in their diets.

At Columbia University College of Physicians and Surgeons, researchers investigated the importance of reducing saturated fat in a cholesterol-lowering diet. They compared the effects of several dietary plans—one that provided 37 percent of calories from fat (including 16 percent from saturated fats), and two comprised of 30 percent fat (one of which provided 14 percent of calories from saturated fats, while the other provided 9 percent from saturated fats). The volunteers who ate the diet with the lowest saturated fat content (9 percent) experienced significant drops in their blood cholesterol level, compared with the two other groups. The study concluded that a decline in dietary fat consumption from 37 to 30 percent did not reduce cholesterol levels— unless cuts in saturated fat accounted for this fat reduction. Thus, the amount of saturated fat, not merely the amount of total fat, is critical for reducing blood cholesterol readings.

Even though dietary cholesterol is not as influential as saturated fats upon blood cholesterol levels, it must be considered a significant factor when consumed in excess. *Dietary cholesterol* is found only in foods of animal origin, most notably egg yolks and organ meats (liver, brain, sweetbreads), as well as the flesh of all animals (beef, pork, lamb, poultry, fish). Some shellfish (such as shrimp) are also high in dietary cholesterol. There is no cholesterol in plant foods, including vegetables, fruits, nuts, and cereals (although some of these items may contain saturated fat).

In spite of the long-recognized contribution of dietary cholesterol to high blood cholesterol, the average American continues to consume an excessive amount. Even though the body manufactures as much cholesterol as it needs, the average American takes in an extra 350 to 450 milligrams per day in his or her food. If you are predisposed toward high blood cholesterol, that's enough to add to your trouble. The National Cholesterol Education Program guidelines recommend a daily cholesterol intake of less than 300 milligrams for the average person. If your blood cholesterol remains high at that level of consumption, the NCEP advises that cholesterol intake be cut further to less than 200 milligrams per day.

Chart 6

SOURCES OF FAT IN YOUR FOOD

Saturated fats: Beef, pork, and lamb
Poultry
Lard
Butter
Egg yolks, milk, cream, and cheese
Coconut and its oil
Palm and palm kernel oils
Vegetable shortening

Polyunsaturated: Corn oil
Cottonseed oil
Sesame oil
Soybean oil
Safflower oil
Sunflower seed oil
Most margarines
Some fish oils (especially cold-water
marine fish such as salmon, mackerel,
herring, and sardines)
Pecans
Mayonnaise
Almonds
Walnuts

Monounsaturated: Peanuts and their oil, and peanut butter
Olives and their oil
Some margarines

By now you should be getting the message: If you want to correct high blood cholesterol, and you are eating anything like the average American, you are going to have to change the way you eat. The message is one that makes some people recoil. After all, eating ranks as one of life's greatest pleasures. But you don't have to sacrifice the joy of eating to follow a cholesterol-lowering program. Later in this book, you'll find a program that will help you lower your cholesterol level without your having to eliminate any single food from your diet. In the upcoming days, you'll discover that breakfast, lunch, and dinner can be not only nourishing and enjoyable, but also powerful weapons against your high blood cholesterol level.

Absorption Factors

Absorption factors help to lower your blood cholesterol level by blocking absorption of substances from the intestines that the body uses to make more cholesterol. These absorption factors include a natural tool known as soluble dietary fiber, as well as prescription medications.

With each passing year, the evidence mounts that dietary fiber has some very unique health-promoting qualities. First of all, foods high in fiber are naturally low in dietary fat and cholesterol. That in itself will help prevent high blood cholesterol, but there is another characteristic of fiber that may be even more important. Fiber seems to have the power to *attract* certain fatty substances in the gastrointestinal tract, escorting them to the stool and out of the body; this prevents the body from using them to manufacture cholesterol in the liver, so your blood cholesterol level goes down. And in addition to this apparent ability to lower the LDL level, some studies suggest that diets high in soluble fiber may also raise the HDL level. As we've noted before, and we'll discuss in more detail soon, this contributes even more to reducing the risk of coronary heart disease.

In 1987, researchers at the University of California, San Diego, discovered the significant effect that fiber can have on heart disease. In their twelve-year study, the dietary patterns of a broad cross-section of 859 men and women (ages 50 to 79) were monitored. In this group, a modest increase in fiber intake of just 6 grams a day (up from an average of 12 grams) reduced the death rate from heart disease by 25 percent in both sexes.

Dietary fiber is found in plant foods. This part of the plant is resistant to the body's digestive-tract enzymes. As a result, only a relatively small amount of fiber is digested or metabolized in the stomach or intestines, most of it moving through the gastrointestinal tract and ending up in your stool. High-fiber diets tend to slow the rate of digestion and food absorption, and they provide a feeling of satiety or a "full" stomach.

There are two general types of plant fiber: insoluble and soluble. Insoluble fiber doesn't dissolve in water. It includes fiber components such as lignin, cellulose, and hemicellulose, which provide plant foods with their firm structure, allowing them to pass through the intestines almost untouched. By contrast, soluble fiber—made up of ingredients such as pectin and guar gum—does dissolve in water. It can be broken down by intestinal bacteria and is the form largely responsible for the positive, cholesterol-lowering effects of fiber. Soluble fiber attaches in the intestines to substances such as bile acids, which can be used by the liver to make more cholesterol, and instead causes them to be eliminated from the body. So while insoluble fiber has many other benefits, you should concentrate on consuming the *soluble* type when your goal is to reduce your cholesterol level.

The richest sources of fiber are vegetables, whole-grain breads and cereals, brown rice, beans and other legumes, and fruits. Within these groups, there are many specific foods that are especially high in the amount of *soluble* fiber they contain, such as kidney or pinto beans, black-eyed peas, and oat bran. That makes these foods especially effective in helping you lower your blood cholesterol level. However, many foods that would seem to be very similar to these, such as wheat bran, lettuce, and spinach, contain primarily *insoluble* fiber. Even though these foods are very high in their total amount of dietary fiber, they are not the best alternatives in their general food groups if lowering blood cholesterol levels is your goal. The charts in Chapter Nine will help you quickly identify foods that are high in soluble fiber.

Absorption factors are more important in cholesterol control than many people realize—perhaps just as significant as reducing your intake of dietary fat and cholesterol. Moderate cutbacks in fat and cholesterol, such as those recommended by the American Heart Association, will lower total cholesterol by 5–15 percent in most people. The Multiple Risk

Factor Intervention Trial reported that individuals who adhere closely to modest cuts in fat and cholesterol experienced an average total cholesterol reduction of 10.5 percent. Modest additions of soluble dietary fiber are capable of creating equally large drops. Put the two strategies together, and you have a program that in many people can lower blood cholesterol levels by 20 percent or more—without any major sacrifice.

If you started with a cholesterol level of 200, adding soluble fiber in addition to lowering your fat intake might get your level to 160 instead of 180. From a starting point of 250, you'd have a good chance of reaching 200 instead of 225. Even if you started with a very high cholesterol level—say 350—working on the absorption factor as well as the intake factor could take your level to 280 instead of 315. As your doctor will tell you, that's a much safer place to be on the risk scale, even if you still need medications to reduce the cholesterol level further.

A study conducted by Dr. David J. A. Jenkins and his colleagues confirmed the importance of high fiber intake in conjunction with a low-fat diet. They evaluated 43 volunteers with high cholesterol levels, placing them on diets that were low in saturated fat and dietary cholesterol, and adding either soluble or insoluble fiber to their meal plans. When the subjects consumed large amounts of soluble fiber (obtained through foods such as peas, beans, oat bran, barley, and dried lentils), their total cholesterol levels declined from an average of 267 to 230, and their LDL cholesterol fell from 180 to 154 by the fourth week of the study. These decreases were larger than those seen on the insoluble fiber-rich, low-fat diet.

In spite of the fact that a wide variety of tasty, attractive, and inexpensive high fiber foods are available, the average American now consumes only about 10 to 15 grams of dietary fiber a day. That's not nearly enough if you have high blood cholesterol, in which case your goal should be two to three times that much. Most of us have a lot of work to do. Fiber is a simple—and inexpensive—food component to add to your diet. And as you will see in Chapter Nine, you can get your fiber from a variety of foods—beans, oat bran, fruits, vegetables, and breads.

By the way, there are some other benefits from a high fiber diet besides lowering your cholesterol level. High fiber foods tend to be more filling in spite of the fact they are relatively low in calories, which makes them ideal for anyone who desires to lose weight. They tend to have a high water content, which—combined with the indigestibility of the fiber itself—relieves and prevents constipation and promotes "regularity" (that's not important medically, but it makes some people feel better). Also, these foods tend to be very rich in vitamins, minerals, and other nutrients, and they provide you with a natural and efficient way to obtain these vital substances.

WHAT DETERMINES YOUR HDL LEVEL?

As you have already learned, not all of the cholesterol in your bloodstream is bad for you. The HDL (high density lipoprotein) cholesterol, actually has a protective effect against coronary heart disease, so the higher your HDL cholesterol level, the better. A number of factors can influence the HDL level:

- *Heredity:* As with cholesterol in general, the HDL portion is influenced by heredity. If you have inherited a tendency toward a high level of HDL, consider yourself fortunate.
- *Exercise*: Physical activity is one of the best ways to raise your HDL level, so if you want to increase it, get your body moving. You don't need to exercise to the point of exhaustion; rather, a program of regular, moderate activity can do it. We'll discuss the relationship between exercise and HDL cholesterol—and how to get started with exercise—in Chapter Ten.
- *Smoking*: Smoking can reduce HDL levels, which is just one of the ways that cigarettes increase the risk of heart attacks. By quitting cigarettes, you can raise your HDL and decrease your chances of a heart attack.
- *Weight*: As your weight goes up, your HDL concentration tends to decline. By losing weight, you can reverse the process. In a study by University of Pennsylvania researchers, published in 1981, a group of men who lost an average of 24 pounds elevated their HDL levels by 5 percent. Though this may not sound like much compared to the percentage decreases that we have been describing for LDL cholesterol, a small increase in HDL cholesterol can make a very significant difference in the risk of heart attacks due to atherosclerosis.

THE DAMAGE CHOLESTEROL PRODUCES

No matter what factors are causing your cholesterol problem, the consequences are the same: Cholesterol and other fatty substances begin accumulating in the walls of your arteries, forming yellowish plaque that narrows down the size of the opening through which blood can flow. Over many years, these deposits can narrow the arteries to the point where they become totally blocked off. The process affects almost all arteries in the body, but the coronary arteries (the arteries that supply blood to the heart) are particularly vulnerable.

Initially, there are no symptoms, so you will have no way of knowing that the arteries are being damaged. As the blockage of blood flow progresses over time, however, and the heart muscle is no longer receiving all the blood and oxygen it needs to function, chest pains (angina pectoris) may begin to occur. This is often the first symptom of the developing disease—a sign that the heart needs more oxygen than it is able to get. But in many people with atherosclerosis, the first sign of trouble is a heart attack—often a fatal one. Atherosclerosis may also contribute to high blood pressure and strokes.

It is hard to understand how atherosclerosis could reach such a severe stage as to jeopardize or cost you your life without an obvious warning, but it often does. So don't wait for such a warning before you take action against all of the risk factors for heart disease. If you've been told that your blood cholesterol is too high, look upon that as a blessing in disguise. Think of it as a gentle warning sign that may save you from experiencing a harsher one.

THE ROLE OF ANTIOXIDANT VITAMINS

In the years ahead, we will learn more about high blood cholesterol, and in turn, perhaps develop new strategies for lowering it. Already, considerable attention is being directed at vitamins E, A, and C—the so-called antioxidant vitamins—and how they may interfere with a process called oxidation that contributes to coronary heart disease and the buildup of plaques in coronary arteries. Researchers believe that as LDL cholesterol becomes oxidized by molecules called free radicals in the body, the LDL causes damage to the walls of the arteries, producing a narrowing of the arteries and a higher risk of heart attacks and other vascular problems. However, antioxidant vitamins could interfere with this process by neutralizing the free radicals.

Perhaps the strongest evidence to date involves vitamin E. Major studies at Harvard University, published in 1993, found an association between the consumption of vitamin E and a reduced risk of coronary heart disease. Women, for instance, who took vitamin E supplements for more than two years had only a little more than half the risk of heart disease as did nonusers of the vitamin. Even women with a prior history of heart attacks, heart bypass surgery, or chest pain have shown a much lower incidence of subsequent heart attacks when they took high levels of antioxidant vitamins.

As yet, however, there is not a proven cause-and-effect relationship between the use of antioxidant vitamins and a reduction in heart disease risk, nor are vitamins a substitute for a poor diet. Nevertheless, in those subjects taking between 100 and 250 I.U. of vitamin E, supplementation appears safe and potentially beneficial. Remember, however, that those persons who took vitamin supplements in the Harvard studies also adopted other health-promoting habits, clouding the issue of the precise effect of vitamin E. If you want to supplement your diet with vitamin E because you think it may lower your risk of heart disease, that's fine—but also incorporate the other *proven* strategies in this book at the same time.

IN CONCLUSION

Fortunately, the scientific evidence is strong for the program we will discuss in this book. You *can* cut your blood cholesterol level by decreasing the amount of fat (especially saturated fat) and cholesterol you eat and by increasing your intake of high fiber foods (especially soluble fiber).

Don't ignore any of the other important risk factors either. If you smoke, quit now. If you have hypertension or diabetes, work closely with your doctor to keep your blood pressure and your blood sugar under control. Lose weight if you need to, and engage in regular exercise. Doing these things will not only reduce your risk of heart disease, but also improve the way you feel and enhance the quality of your life.

4

♥　♥　♥　♥

TOTAL CHOLESTEROL
How High Is Too High?

The risk of developing heart disease actually begins to rise after the blood cholesterol level exceeds about 140, but initially this increase in risk is slight. The higher the cholesterol rises, the more rapidly the cardiovascular risk increases. A cholesterol level of 200 raises the heart attack risk about 50 percent over a level of 150. But the next 50 points have a much more dramatic effect. A cholesterol level of 250 increases the heart attack risk by about three times over the 150 figure. (You can see this graphically in Chart 4, on page 15).

At what level should you become concerned enough to start a cholesterol-lowering program? The answer to that question has changed greatly during the last few years. In a 1983 survey of 412 cardiologists, 31 percent of the doctors said that a patient's cholesterol level would have to be 300 or higher before they would start dietary therapy. *None* of the doctors who participated in that study said he would recommend dietary treatment for patients with cholesterol levels of 240 or less.

By 1986, when a similar group of 318 heart specialists was asked the same question, the situation had changed dramatically. Only 5 percent of the doctors said they would wait to initiate dietary therapy until the cholesterol level reached 300, and 54 percent reported that they began dietary treatment of their patients at levels of 240 or lower.

In 1987, the National Cholesterol Education Program convened an expert panel to establish clear guidelines that physicians could use for making these decisions. The panel's report (referred to earlier) provided both doctors and the general public with a uniform plan for deciding when special cholesterol testing and therapy were necessary. The report was updated in 1993, and its general guidelines are as follows:

Total Blood Cholesterol
Less than 200 mg/dl = desirable blood cholesterol
200-239 mg/dl = borderline-high blood cholesterol
240 mg/dl or more = high blood cholesterol

LDL Cholesterol
Less than 130 mg/dl = desirable LDL cholesterol
130-159 mg/dl = borderline high-risk LDL cholesterol
160 mg/dl or more = high-risk LDL cholesterol

HDL Cholesterol
Less than 35 mg/dl = low HDL cholesterol

How did the experts arrive at these clear-cut dividing lines between "desirable," "borderline," and "high-risk" levels? Their decision had to be somewhat arbitrary, since the risk of heart disease goes up continually as the total cholesterol and the LDL cholesterol levels rise above certain levels, but they justified these "cut-points" because they are the approximate levels at which the risk of heart disease begins to rise more steeply.

The panel recommended that all adults twenty years of age and older should have their *total blood cholesterol* level measured at least once every five years. They recommended this particular blood test for screening because it is widely available, easy to perform, relatively inexpensive, and it can be performed in a nonfasting state. The report also advised an HDL cholesterol test at the same time, as long as an accurate measurement could be ensured. For individuals already diagnosed with coronary heart disease, the panel recommended that screenings include measurements of not only total and HDL cholesterol levels, but also LDL and triglyceride values.

Depending on the outcomes of these tests—and whether you already have evidence of coronary heart disease and/or its risk factors—your doctor may provide additional evaluation, guidance, or treatment. This may include additional testing in the future, an exercise program, dietary changes, and modification of your risk factors. If your cholesterol remains high despite non-drug therapy, your doctor may consider drug treatment.

When these guidelines were first released, a major educational effort was organized by the National Institutes of Health and leading medical organizations to quickly inform American physicians about the guidelines and urge their adoption. The doctors were ready and willing. For the first time, they had some precise recommendations that could easily be understood and carried out by patients. The guidelines received widespread publicity in the consumer press, too. As a result, many people

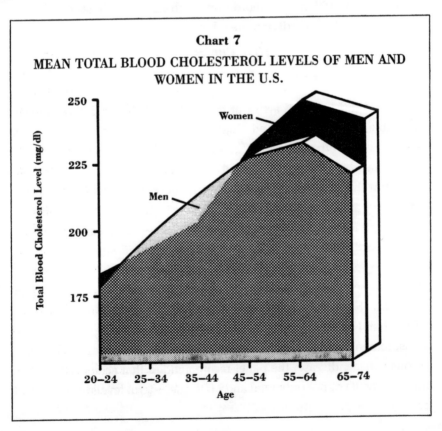

Chart 7

MEAN TOTAL BLOOD CHOLESTEROL LEVELS OF MEN AND WOMEN IN THE U.S.

who had previously ignored the issue of cholesterol or been confused by it now became personally interested and involved. A large number of people wanted to "know their number," and find out what their risks were. Physicians began to offer cholesterol screening tests during routine visits, and more patients began to take advantage of them. Public screening programs sprang up across the country, and people lined up at shopping malls and health fairs to get their fingers pricked. Before long, cholesterol became a "hot" topic, and millions more Americans could say they knew their own number.

Initial reports from these screening programs reveal that the problem of high blood cholesterol is widespread and serious. About 50 percent of the people screened have cholesterol levels above 200. Of this group, approximately half have cholesterol levels over 240. That means that one-quarter of all American adults have cholesterol levels that greatly increase their risk of coronary heart disease.

In addition to stimulating interest in the subject of cholesterol, the guidelines have been valuable in many other ways. They have provided doctors with consistent answers to the many questions that patients ask, and they have created a reasonable standard for evaluating way cholesterol problems are handled. Also, the availability of these understandable guidelines has motivated many people to make healthful dietary changes that might otherwise have been skipped.

It was the precision and clarity of the guidelines that made them so useful and resulted in their wide dissemination and use. But as you and your doctor use them, there are some important points to keep in mind. For instance, the term "desirable" was used to describe blood cholesterol levels up to 199; while 199 may be desirable when compared to a level of 240, it still results in a significantly higher risk of coronary heart disease than does a level of 160. The fact is, most Americans with blood cholesterol levels of 190 could easily reduce their levels to 160 or lower, simply by changing their diets. That would significantly lower their risk of subsequent heart attacks. So don't let the "desirable" label discourage you from making changes that can reduce your cholesterol level even further.

Also, bear in mind that the risk related to cholesterol increases continuously as the cholesterol level rises. By following the guidelines stringently, one person whose blood cholesterol is 201 may be told that he has

---

Chart 8

RISK FACTORS FOR CORONARY HEART DISEASE
(other than high blood cholesterol)

Age: Men age 45 and over; women, age 55 and over (or premature menopause without estrogen replacement therapy)

High blood pressure

Cigarette smoking

Family history of premature coronary heart disease (definite heart attack or sudden death before age 55 in father or other male first-degree relative, or before age 65 in mother or other female first-degree relative)

Diabetes

Low HDL cholesterol level: HDL less than 35 mg/dl, confirmed by repeat measurement

---

a "borderline-high" level, while another person whose result is 199 is told that his cholesterol level is "desirable." Because the readings of these individuals are so close, many doctors will personalize their recommendations based not solely on the guidelines, but also on each patient's own circumstances (for instance, whether they have other risk factors for heart disease, such as smoking or high blood pressure).

The same situation might occur at the higher dividing line. Under the expert panel's guidelines, a person whose cholesterol level is 239 is in the borderline-high zone, while another person with a level of 241 has a high reading. That information may be reassuring to the person with the lower level and extremely frightening for the person with the higher value—when, in reality, their risks regarding cholesterol are almost identical.

The recommendations, then, are simply guidelines. They are not absolutes, and when using them, your doctor will probably make adjustments for factors such as age, sex, heredity, and lifestyle. As Chart 7 demonstrates, cholesterol levels tend to climb with age, and average levels differ between men and women. Blood cholesterol levels begin to rise around the age of twenty, with women's levels slightly lower than men's until the age of menopause. After the menopause, women's cholesterol levels rise considerably higher, while in men they tend to level off. As a result, in their later years many women end up with higher total cholesterol levels than men.

So don't overlook the factors of age and sex. For example, a cholesterol measurement of 190 could be considered desirable in a middle-aged adult, but must be viewed with concern in a child. And a level of 210—certainly higher than it should be in a twenty-year-old—may not be a cause for concern in a seventy-five-year-old.

HOW HIGH IS TOO HIGH FOR YOU?

All other things being equal, the lower your blood cholesterol level, the lower your risk of heart disease. Therefore, any number higher than the one you can *reasonably* achieve with a healthy lifestyle is a number that is too high for you. No matter what cholesterol group you fall into under the guidelines, you should try to get your cholesterol level even lower, as long as it can *reasonably* be done.

Please note the use of the word "reasonably" rather than "possibly." With prescription medications, it is *possible* for almost anyone to reduce his or her blood cholesterol level dramatically—far more than can be achieved with a prudent diet alone. However, the use of drugs cannot be justified in a person whose blood cholesterol level is 201, because the potential risks do not justify the potential benefits. The table turns, however, in someone who cannot get his cholesterol level lower than 250 with diet and exercise alone. In this case, the potential gain with drugs (a 30–70 percent reduction in the risk of heart attack or death as the result of coronary heart disease) may well be worth the cost and risks of taking medication.

It becomes even more important to lower your cholesterol level if you have any of the other risk factors for coronary heart disease (see Chart 8). Having two or more risk factors at the same time increases the danger enormously. For example, if your cholesterol level is over 240 and you also have high blood pressure, your risk of heart disease may increase six-fold. If, in addition, you smoke, your risk could increase more than twenty times. (The best way to reduce such "combination risks" is to quit smoking and work with your physician to control your blood pressure.)

This book will help you determine what your own ideal blood cholesterol level should be and what alternatives are available for helping you reach that level. Before you decide what therapy is necessary or appropriate, it is important that you discuss these questions with your physician. No matter what your blood cholesterol level, your physician can be a valuable partner in your efforts to control it. The doctor can also tell you about the potential costs, risks, and benefits of each alternative. Take advantage of this opportunity to work with your doctor this way. With cholesterol— as with any health concern—you want all the help you can get.

5

♥　♥　♥　♥

HDL CHOLESTEROL
How Low Is Too Low?

While lowering your *total* cholesterol is a good idea, it is important to remember that high-density lipoproteins (HDL, or HDL cholesterol) require a different strategy. As you have learned, HDL is one form of cholesterol on which you want to count upward, because it helps to remove cholesterol from the body and can actually prevent the buildup of cholesterol in the walls of your arteries.

HDL cholesterol levels are determined in significant part by your heredity. They are also influenced by your age and sex. In children, HDL levels are essentially the same in boys and girls. Around puberty, HDL levels drop about 20 percent in the boys, and they remain lower in men than in women throughout adult life.

It is more difficult to raise your HDL level than it is to lower your total cholesterol level. Diet can affect HDL levels, but in most studies, not nearly as much as it affects LDLs. A high-carbohydrate, low-fat diet will lower LDLs as much as 15 percent but is not likely to raise your HDL levels as much—although not all studies agree with this finding. Some researchers have reported that as total cholesterol declines markedly, HDL readings decrease as well—an odd and unwelcome paradox for people attempting to improve their cardiovascular health. (An editorial in the *New England Journal of Medicine* by Harvard Medical School investigators described a typical scenario in which adoption of a low-fat diet produced decreases in total cholesterol from 260 to 210, but declines in HDL readings from 40 to 32.)

Fortunately, however, strategies are available for maintaining high HDL levels. They can be raised significantly by exercise, a moderate intake of alcoholic beverages (some doctors feel that the kind of HDL raised by alcohol is not as helpful as that raised by regular exercise), and leanness. (We'll discuss each of these approaches in more detail in Chapter Ten.) By contrast, HDL levels are lowered (and your risk of heart disease increased) by cigarette smoking, sedentary behavior, obesity, and diabetes. (We will discuss some of these issues and relevant studies later.) And when it comes to diet, many authorities suggest that most dietary

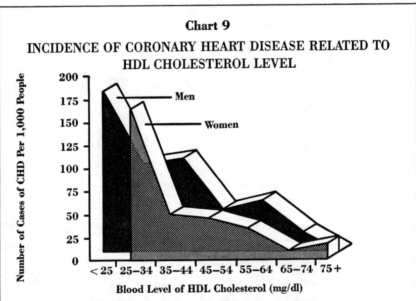

Chart 9

INCIDENCE OF CORONARY HEART DISEASE RELATED TO HDL CHOLESTEROL LEVEL

Number of Cases of CHD Per 1,000 People

Blood Level of HDL Cholesterol (mg/dl)

This chart from the Framingham Heart Study relates the incidence of coronary heart disease (per 1,000 men and women) to the HDL cholesterol level. In both sexes, as HDL levels rose, the rate of heart disease declined. For instance, while 175 (of 1,000) men with an HDL cholesterol reading below 25 had coronary heart disease, that figure fell to 50 among men with HDL values between 45 and 54.

fats should be monounsaturates (such as olive oil), since polyunsaturates, especially in high amounts, tend to reduce HDL levels.

HDL'S PROTECTIVE EFFECT

As we mentioned earlier, the concentration of HDL cholesterol is *inversely* related to the development of coronary heart disease. In other words, people with very high levels of HDLs have a much lower than average risk of heart disease, while those with very low levels have a higher than average risk. Chart 9, based on research in Framingham, Massachusetts, reveals just how dramatic the protective effect of HDL cholesterol can be. Among the people who were studied in Framingham (men and women aged 50 to 80), those with HDL cholesterol levels below 35 suffered heart disease eight times more often than those whose HDL levels were 65 and over.

HOW HIGH IS HIGH ENOUGH?

The Framingham researchers measured the protective effect of different HDL levels on the rate of heart attacks by studying both healthy people and people who had one or more risk factors for heart disease (such as high total blood cholesterol, high blood pressure, cigarette use, or abnormal electrocardiograms). They divided all these people into groups based not only on the risk factors, but also on their HDL cholesterol levels. By measuring what happened to people at each HDL level, they were able to come up with a series of "multipliers" that objectively measured the protective effect of high HDL (or the increased risk that accompanies a very low HDL level). These multipliers are shown in Chart 10.

No matter what your present risk of coronary heart disease, increasing your HDL level will help lower it. High HDL levels can even help you overcome, at least in part, the increased risk of an elevated *total* cholesterol level. In fact, some people with high total cholesterol levels have HDL levels that are also very high—sometimes high enough to completely counterbalance the increased risk of the high total cholesterol. For example, a person who has a total blood cholesterol level of 210 with an HDL of 70 probably has a *lower* risk of heart disease than a person whose total cholesterol level is 200 with an HDL of only 50. Needless to say, the higher you get your HDL level, the more protection you have against heart disease.

Chart 10

**THE EFFECT OF HDL LEVELS ON THE RISK
OF CORONARY HEART DISEASE**

HDL Level (mg/dl)	Multiplier for Men	Multiplier for Women
30	1.82	—
35	1.49	—
40	1.22	1.94
45	1.00	1.55
50	0.82	1.25
55	0.67	1.00
60	0.55	0.80
65	0.45	0.64
70	—	0.52
75	—	—

The average HDL cholesterol level is 45 for American men and 55 for American women. Since those levels—by definition—will produce an average risk, they are assigned a multiplier value of 1.00. As the HDL level increases, the risk of coronary heart disease drops, and the numerical value of the multiplier goes down. For example, if you are a man and your HDL cholesterol level goes up from 45 to 60, your risk at the new level is only .55 times (55 percent) what it was at the original level. If your HDL level goes down from 45 to 35, your risk of coronary heart disease goes up 1.49 times (49 percent).

THE TOTAL CHOLESTEROL/HDL (TC/HDL) RATIO

If your doctor follows the National Cholesterol Education Program guidelines, he or she will measure both your total and HDL cholesterol levels. With that information in hand, the significance of your HDL level can be estimated—particularly the role it plays in your risk of heart disease—by calculating the ratio between your total cholesterol level and your HDL cholesterol level (the total cholesterol/HDL, or TC/HDL, ratio). For example:

$$\text{If your total cholesterol} = 200 \text{ mg/dl}$$
$$\text{and your HDL cholesterol} = 50 \text{ mg/dl}$$
$$\text{your TC/HDL ratio} = \frac{200}{50} = 4.0$$

The TC/HDL ratio shows you in a mathematical way approximately how much more LDL than HDL is present in your blood (remember, in an average person, about 60–70 percent of the total cholesterol in the blood is in the form of LDLs). The more LDL you have in relation to the HDL present, the higher your ratio will be and the higher your risk will be. The less LDL in relation to the HDL present, the lower your ratio and risk will be. These can be clarified by the following two examples:

If your total cholesterol went up and your HDL stayed the same, your total cholesterol/HDL ratio would be higher and your risk would be higher than in the example above:

$$\text{If your total cholesterol} = 250 \text{ mg/dl}$$
$$\text{and your HDL cholesterol} = 50 \text{ mg/dl}$$
$$\text{your TC/HDL ratio} = \frac{250}{50} = 5.0$$

If your HDL went up and your total cholesterol stayed the same, your total cholesterol/HDL ratio and your risk of coronary heart disease are lower than in the initial example:

$$\text{If your total cholesterol} = 200 \text{ mg/dl}$$
$$\text{and your HDL cholesterol} = 60 \text{ mg/dl}$$
$$\text{your TC/HDL ratio} = \frac{200}{60} = 3.33$$

HOW LOW IS LOW ENOUGH FOR THE TC/HDL RATIO?

The average American male has a total cholesterol/HDL ratio of 4.5. In American women, the average ratio is 4.0. (This accounts, at least in part, for the fact that American females have a lower rate of heart disease than males). But average isn't good enough—the healthiest possible ratio you can *reasonably* achieve is the one you should be seeking.

You can improve (lower) your TC/HDL ratio two ways:

1. Lower your LDL cholesterol level.
2. Raise your HDL level.

You really should try to do both. Changing either one in the right direction will improve your TC/HDL ratio, and changing both will produce dramatic results. You will learn how to accomplish this in Part Two.

While your cholesterol ratio is a good summary of your overall risk of heart disease, make sure you know and understand each of your cholesterol measurements, too. And though there are no guarantees that you will be able to get your HDL level up or your TC/HDL ratio down by using this program, any progress you make toward those goals will mean you have reduced your risk of heart problems and increased your chances for a healthy life. That's worth at least thirty days of your time and attention, isn't it?

6

♥　♥　♥　♥

WHAT'S YOUR CHOLESTEROL NUMBER?

It is impossible to count out cholesterol accurately if you don't know where to start counting. That is why a major campaign was recently launched to get you to "know your number"—the number that represents your total blood cholesterol level. In spite of the obvious value of knowing your number, a surprisingly small percentage of Americans are familiar with theirs. A 1986 survey in thirty-three states and the District of Columbia revealed that only about half of those surveyed had ever had their blood cholesterol measured. Of the half that had been tested, only 8 percent had been told by their doctors that their blood cholesterol level was high, and only 7 percent of the tested half knew their actual levels.

But the tide is turning now, and many more people are being tested and learning their results. In part, this increased interest is due to the NCEP expert panel's report, which recommended that every adult age twenty or over be tested at least every five years. By following this advice, you can ensure that if your blood cholesterol rises to high levels, you will be treated before it has much of an opportunity to damage your blood vessels.

There are real benefits to knowing your blood cholesterol level early in adult life. It enables you to recognize any upward trend that develops as you grow older, so you can take corrective measures *before* your blood cholesterol reaches the high-risk zone. These tests may also help to uncover inherited tendencies toward high cholesterol levels, providing clues that can help your entire family get the treatment they need before major damage occurs.

WHO SHOULD BE TESTED AND HOW OFTEN?

The ideal time to have your blood cholesterol measured is when you are in the doctor's office for a routine visit. It takes just a few minutes, adds relatively little to the cost of the visit, and gives you an opportunity to discuss this important subject with your physician. So if you are seeing your doctor and have not had your cholesterol measured in the last five years, talk to him or her about having the test done at that time. If you are pregnant or quite ill, the doctor may prefer to wait a while before testing you. (This will be explained later in this chapter.) If you are not due for a regular checkup and have no medical problems that are likely to bring you to the doctor in the near future, you can probably make arrangements for a brief visit just to have blood drawn for a cholesterol test. For a review of the NCEP panel's guidelines on cholesterol testing, see page 39.

Since the development of small, portable analyzers that can measure blood cholesterol levels almost anywhere, many opportunities for cholesterol screening are now available outside the doctor's office. Most of these screening programs offer the advantages of convenience and very low cost, although their accuracy and value have been questioned by some experts. If you undergo such a test, it is important that you discuss the meaning of the results with your doctor. This is especially important if your total cholesterol is over 200.

Cholesterol Testing for Children

In 1992, the Expert Panel on Blood Cholesterol Levels in Children and Adolescents established guidelines specifically for children, including recommendations for cholesterol testing. As the chart below shows, the panel concluded that healthy children should have substantially lower cholesterol levels than adults (e.g., while total cholesterol between 200 and 239 is considered "borderline" in adults, these same values are "high" when they occur in children with a family history of high cholesterol or early cardiovascular problems). The experts emphasized that the process leading to blocked arteries starts in childhood and is influenced by high blood cholesterol levels.

TOTAL CHOLESTEROL LEVELS IN CHILDREN & ADOLESCENTS FROM FAMILIES WITH HIGH CHOLESTEROL LEVELS OR EARLY CARDIOVASCULAR DISEASE		
Acceptable	*Borderline*	*High*
Less than 170	170–199	200 and over

However, the panel did *not* recommend that *all* children undergo routine cholesterol testing. Instead, it advised that the cholesterol levels for only those at highest risk be monitored. These include children and adolescents whose parents or grandparents fall into one or more of the following categories:

- At age 55 or less, they underwent diagnostic coronary arteriography, and were found to have coronary atherosclerosis. This includes individuals who have undergone coronary bypass surgery or balloon angioplasty.
- At age 55 or less, they had a heart attack, angina (chest pain), stroke, peripheral vascular disease, or sudden cardiac death.
- They have high blood cholesterol (240 mg/dl or more).

In addition to a cholesterol test, those children with a family history of coronary heart disease will require a complete lipoprotein profile. For example, in those families with an inherited low HDL, a single cholesterol test would not detect this problem. A doctor might also recommend testing for children who fall into other categories, such as adolescents who are at higher risk for coronary heart disease because they smoke cigarettes, have high blood pressure, are overweight, and/or have excessive amounts of saturated fat, total fat, and cholesterol in their diets.

WHAT TESTS ARE AVAILABLE?

To measure your blood cholesterol, your doctor or a technician will draw a small blood sample for analysis. If the analysis is done immediately with a blood analyzer in the doctor's office or at a community screening site, a simple fingerstick will usually suffice to produce the few drops of blood that are necessary. If the specimen is sent out to a laboratory for analysis, a larger specimen is usually taken from a vein.

Several different tests are currently being used to measure blood levels of cholesterol and other substances related to cardiovascular risk, the most common ones being the "total blood cholesterol" test and a group of tests known as "lipoprotein analysis" (also referred to as a "lipid profile"). The total blood cholesterol test provides a single number that includes all the measurable cholesterol in your blood. This includes HDL (the so-called good cholesterol), LDL (the so-called bad cholesterol), and VLDL (which carries triglycerides or blood fats through the body). By contrast, the lipid profile is really several tests that separately report your blood HDL, LDL, triglycerides, and total cholesterol level.

Total Blood Cholesterol

There are some advantages to the total blood cholesterol test. It can be done easily, it is widely available, and you do not have to fast before the blood is drawn. Also, it is the least expensive test for measuring cholesterol, with a cost ranging from about $5 to $15, depending on where the test is done. For these reasons, the total blood cholesterol test is a good test for screening at least once every five years for those individuals with desirable cholesterol levels. (As we've mentioned earlier, the NCEP also now recommends an HDL test at the same time.)

However, there are limitations to the value of the total cholesterol test, including the possibility of an inaccurate result. Though modern analyzers have reduced this risk to a minimum and most such errors are small, the chance of an inaccurate measurement must always be kept in mind. In rare cases, the error may be very large, but this possibility is not unique to the total blood cholesterol test; the same problem exists—to a greater or lesser degree—for many medical tests that are done today.

Another weakness of the total cholesterol test is its inability to reveal how much of the total cholesterol is made up of LDL cholesterol and how much consists of HDL. Two people who have the same total choles-terol level may have quite different risks of coronary heart disease if the amounts of HDL in their blood differ greatly. For example, if two people have identical total cholesterol levels of 220, but one has an HDL level of 55 while the other has an HDL level of 35, the first person will have a significantly lower risk of coronary heart disease than the second. The only way to determine this difference between these two individuals is by performing an HDL test along with the total cholesterol measurement or by getting the even more complete lipid profile.

For all these reasons, decisions about treating high blood cholesterol should not be made on the basis of a single test that shows an elevated total blood cholesterol. In Chapter Four, we described the National Cholesterol Education Program's recommendations which include obtain-ing an HDL reading—along with a total cholesterol value—as part of the screening. If you need to, go back and review these guidelines. They should be the ones your doctor uses in scheduling your own blood cho-lesterol tests.

Lipoprotein Analysis (The Lipid Profile)

As you have learned, the lipoprotein analysis provides much more infor-mation about the nature of the cholesterol in your body than a total blood cholesterol measurement, but it is not used for routine screening because it is more expensive (approximately $35 to $50, depending on where you get tested) and somewhat more inconvenient (you must fast for twelve hours before the blood sample is drawn). For this test it is usually necessary to take a blood sample from your vein for analysis at a laboratory, although some labs and screening centers are equipped to perform these tests on a fingerstick specimen.

Some physicians prefer to order the lipid profile for the initial screening, since it provides so much more information and it identifies people whose risk is unusually high because their ratio of total cholesterol to HDL is unfavorable. The lipid profile may also be appropriate for people who have a strong family history of heart disease or who have close relatives with severely elevated cholesterol levels.

The National Cholesterol Education Program recommends that the lipoprotein analysis be repeated at regular intervals in people whose cholesterol problems are severe enough to require drug therapy, although measurement of the total cholesterol level alone may be sufficient for these people at most medical checkups.

Keep in mind, however, that HDL measurements in particular often lack the accuracy necessary to be useful to you and your doctor. Studies indicate that some methods of assessing HDL values produce lower measurements than others. Also, the handling and storage of blood samples before analysis can influence the accuracy of the reading. Ask your doctor about the quality-control methods used at the laboratory that performs evaluations on the samples from his patients.

OTHER FACTORS THAT AFFECT THE MEASUREMENT OF YOUR CHOLESTEROL LEVEL

Anyone who has had a cholesterol measurement taken more than once in a relatively short period of time (within a few days, a few hours, or even a few minutes) knows that you rarely get the same number twice. This happens because of various factors that can affect the test results, including the following:

- The accuracy of the particular instrument used to perform the analysis
- The use of different instruments
- Quality-control measures

- Human error
- Biological variability (including the effect of season of the year, nutritional status, and the position of the body when the blood was drawn)
- Your medical condition and the medications you are taking

Any one of these factors can influence the results of a total blood cholesterol test or lipoprotein analysis upward or downward. If two or more factors are operating at the same time, there can be an even greater difference between the results of two tests performed on the same person within a relatively short period of time. It is important to be aware that test results can vary this way—not to discourage you from having your blood cholesterol measured, but so that you will interpret the results of any single test with caution.

Accuracy of the Analyzer Instrument

The most accurate cholesterol measurements in the United States (probably in the world) are done in a group of federally funded reference laboratories that employ extremely precise methods that are just not practical for everyday lab use. These special laboratories set the standard of accuracy against which all other labs and all analyzing instruments are compared. The laboratories and analyzers that will be measuring your cholesterol levels and lipid profiles are considered acceptably accurate if the answers they produce are within 5 percent of the results that would have been obtained if your blood specimen had been analyzed in one of the reference labs.

In simple terms, that means that if your total blood cholesterol level is actually 200, an analyzer or laboratory may produce results anywhere between 190 and 210—and be considered acceptably accurate. If your blood is tested five times within five minutes on the same analyzer, you may get results of 190, 195, 200, 205, and 210, and the machine will be considered to be performing within the expected range of accuracy.

Yet if you recall the guidelines established by the National Cholesterol Education Program, two of those results would have placed you in the "desirable" blood cholesterol range (under 200), while three would have fallen into the "borderline-high" zone. If ever there was a reason not to get overly worried (or overly confident) about a single blood cholesterol reading, this is it. That's also why a second, confirming test is recommended whenever the first test shows your cholesterol level to be higher than the desirable range. A second test is not considered necessary if the first one places you in the desirable range.

Using Different Analyzer Instruments

Each analyzer instrument is calibrated at the factory to operate within the range of accuracy just described. However, one instrument may produce test results that are consistently higher than those of another. For example, if five specimens of blood with actual cholesterol levels of 200 are tested on two analyzers, one of the instruments may report all the levels around 205, while the other may report them all near 195. If you alternated instruments while testing yourself, it could appear as though your blood cholesterol level were changing, when it really was the same. Because of this possibility, if you require (or desire) repeated measurements of your blood cholesterol level, it makes sense to have all of the analyses performed on the same instrument.

Incidentally, the accuracy of a cholesterol-measuring analyzer does not necessarily increase with its price. Several portable cholesterol analyzers with price tags under $5,000 are producing results comparable to large laboratory analyzers costing more than $150,000. The issues of quality-control procedures and human error are at least as important as the machine being used.

Quality-Control Measures

The analyzers used to measure blood cholesterol levels use space age technology to produce accurate results within minutes. However, these analyzers are extremely delicate instruments, and their day-to-day—even hour-to-hour—accuracy can be affected by such things as power surges and variations in room temperature. To prevent inaccurate readings caused by such factors, most instrument manufacturers recommend that a series of quality-control procedures be performed according to a very precise schedule. Usually, these procedures include recalibrating the analyzer at least once before it is used each day and then again after any incident that could throw off the accuracy of the instrument.

Most large laboratories (including those in hospitals) are required by state laws to keep records of all quality-control measures, and they are inspected at regular intervals to ensure that the regulations are followed. However, sixteen states have no such laws, and in most states that do have them, they are not applied to tests performed in doctors' offices or at community screening projects. If you have any question about the quality-control procedures being used on the instrument that measures your blood cholesterol, ask the person taking your blood specimen or operating the device.

Human Error

One of best features of modern laboratory analyzers is that they are so highly automated, they reduce the likelihood of inaccurate results because of human error. However, there is plenty of room for error before the specimen is inserted into the analyzer. Using just a fraction of a drop of blood too much or too little can throw off results considerably. There is room for human error in all phases of cholesterol testing, from community screening programs to doctors' offices to major reference laboratories. Errors are most likely to occur when untrained personnel are operating the analyzer instruments and when the volume of tests is too great for the resources available, as can occur when mass screening programs are conducted. But the same kinds of errors can take place in the finest laboratories staffed by the most highly qualified people, so the result of any single cholesterol test must be interpreted with caution.

Biological Variability

One of the most important influences upon the results of your cholesterol test is a factor known as biological variability. This refers to the changes that are going on in your body from hour to hour and from day to day, some of which can significantly affect the amount of cholesterol

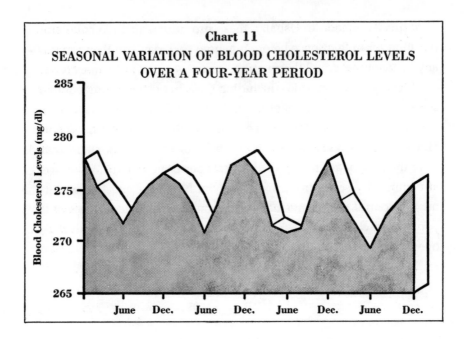

Chart 11

SEASONAL VARIATION OF BLOOD CHOLESTEROL LEVELS
OVER A FOUR-YEAR PERIOD

in your blood. In one study, researchers tested the blood of 22 subjects every hour from 9 A.M. to 5 P.M. and found that these individuals had hourly variations that deviated 2 to 8.6 percent from their mean levels for the day. For example, one person in this study had the following results on nine tests performed at hourly intervals during the same day: 244, 202, 228, 244, 198, 231, 225, 199, and 234. The researchers found no relationship between the cholesterol variations in these subjects and the meals they ate or their activity, and there was no particular time of day when cholesterol levels tended to be higher or lower.

The same researchers tested blood samples from three subjects in this group on several different days after they had fasted overnight, and found great variability from day to day. In one individual, the total *fasting* blood cholesterol levels on five consecutive days were 212, 231, 198, 230, and 249. The levels in these three people were significantly lower when they were measured after fasting than under usual conditions. But other studies suggest that fasting overnight will not lower your total blood cholesterol level more than 1 or 2 percent (although it can definitely affect the level of other fats in the blood, such as triglycerides).

The seasons appear to exert a remarkable effect on blood cholesterol. In one study, in which more than 1,400 men were tested at bimonthly intervals over several years, the average total blood cholesterol level was 7.4 points higher on December 30 than on June 30. Researchers noted the same seasonal variation at all twelve sites in the U.S. where the measurements were taken, although the differences tended to be slightly greater in the southern locations. This seasonal variation could not be explained by dietary changes, weight gain or loss, or whether the subjects had high or low cholesterol levels.

A separate study published in 1992 reached similar conclusions in both men and women. An international research team from the University of Minnesota and the University of Lund in Sweden analyzed cholesterol levels in 3,377 men and 3,900 women, and found the highest values in winter, and the lowest in summer. In women, differences in average total cholesterol levels between the highest and lowest months were 29 points; in men, they were 27 points.

Your cholesterol test can also be affected by the physical position you are in when your blood is drawn. The result will tend to be lower (by as much as 6 percent) if the blood is drawn while you are sitting rather than standing. For this reason, the National Cholesterol Education

---

SHOULD YOU TEST YOUR CHOLESTEROL AT HOME?

In 1993, the first home cholesterol test received approval by the Food and Drug Administration. Available in drugstores without a prescription, the home test requires the user to prick his finger, and place a few drops of blood into a small container in which there is also a test strip. In a few minutes, the strip begins to change colors, and the ultimate length of the colored portion of the strip will help determine (with the assistance of a conversion chart) the individual's blood cholesterol level.

Critics of the home test, however, have raised a number of concerns. They worry about the accuracy of the test, and that it measures only total cholesterol, not HDL or LDL parameters. They also point out that without a doctor present to explain the test results, some individuals may be confused by or misinterpret these findings.

On balance, you are much better off—in terms of accuracy and proper interpretation of the results—to get your cholesterol test at your doctor's office.

Program recommends that specimens for cholesterol tests be taken after you have been in the sitting position for at least five minutes. Also, if a tourniquet is used for drawing blood from a vein, it should be left tightened for as short a time as possible; if it remains on for longer than two minutes, the test result may come back artificially elevated.

Your Medical Condition and the Medications You Are Taking

Your doctor may suggest delaying a cholesterol test if you are pregnant or acutely ill, or if you have suffered a heart attack, stroke, or major trauma (including an operation) within the last three months. That is because all of these conditions can significantly alter the result from what it would be under normal conditions. Here is how some common conditions affect blood cholesterol levels:

- A recent heart attack or stroke may lower your total blood cholesterol by up to 25 percent from its usual level. Severe trauma, including surgery, can produce the same effect.

- Total cholesterol levels will rise gradually throughout pregnancy, until—near full term—they may be 45 percent higher than in the nonpregnant state. It may take up to three months after delivery for them to return to normal.

- Total cholesterol levels and/or HDL levels may be affected by the use of certain medications. Oral contraceptives may raise the total blood cholesterol slightly, while estrogens will raise just the HDL portion. A group of drugs known as beta-blockers, which are used to treat cardiovascular conditions, have been reported to lower HDL levels, as have androgenic steroid drugs (male hormones) and progesterone-like drugs (female hormones). Your physician should be familiar with the effects of various drugs on cholesterol levels. If you have an elevated blood cholesterol reading, he or she will take this factor into account when prescribing medication for you.

NOW YOU KNOW YOUR NUMBER, BUT CAN YOU TRUST IT?

After reading about all the possible opportunities for error in measuring your blood cholesterol level, you might be tempted to ask if it is worth being measured at all. That is a fair question, and the answer requires a measure of faith and a degree of skepticism. Cholesterol tests *are* worth doing, because, even with all their weaknesses, they provide a simple and convenient way to identify one of the most important—and treatable—risk factors for coronary heart disease. Despite the opportunities for error, the vast majority of cholesterol tests are accurate enough to help guide your decisions wisely, and multiple measurements can always be performed.

You will find your total cholesterol test results valuable if you use them as a *general* estimate of your cholesterol-related risk rather than as a precise measure of your cholesterol level. If you are clearly at one of the extremes—for example, 120 or 360—you can be pretty sure (never 100 percent, though) that you are in the clear or have a problem, depending on which end of the scale you fall into. Also, the picture will not change if you are on one of the dividing lines—that is, it really doesn't matter if your cholesterol is 239 or 241, since either level is too high and demands your immediate attention. Similarly, there is no *real* difference between 199 and 201; starting at either level, you may be able to lower your cholesterol to 170 or even lower—and the sooner you do it, the better. On the other hand, if the test says your cholesterol level is 140, relax and enjoy your good health.

If you have questions or concerns about the results of your cholesterol test, discuss them with your physician, who will know if any medical factors could be affecting your test results. He or she can order additional tests, if necessary, or give you advice specifically tailored to your needs.

PART II

♥ ♥ ♥ ♥

COUNTING OUT

7

♥   ♥   ♥   ♥

STARTING THE COUNT

Using Your SF Numbers

Chart 12

NATIONAL CHOLESTEROL EDUCATION PROGRAM
GUIDELINES FOR REDUCING BLOOD CHOLESTEROL LEVEL

- Eat less than 300 milligrams of dietary cholesterol each day (the average American eats about 350 to 450).
- Less than 30 percent of your total daily calories should come from fat (the average American diet is about 35 to 40 percent fat).
- Less than 10 percent of your calories should come from saturated fat (15 to 20 percent of the average American's calories come from saturated fat).
- Choose foods high in complex carbohydrates (fiber and starch).
- Adjust your caloric intake to achieve or maintain a desirable weight.

Like most Americans, you have probably seen or heard these guidelines for lowering your blood cholesterol many times, but are you following them? You will probably have difficulty answering that question. How do you know what percentage of your calories is coming from fat when you can't even tell how many calories you are eating each day? How do you know if you're consuming enough fiber when there's seemingly no way to know how much fiber most foods contain? Until now, to follow the dietary guidelines for controlling cholesterol, you almost had to carry an encyclopedia, a scale, and a computer with you. But not any more, because we have developed a simple series of charts that will do the work and the calculations for you. These charts form the basis for much of the rest of this book. Let's set the stage for what you will find in the following chapters.

In Chapter Eight, there are charts that can help you gain control over saturated fat—a major factor in determining your blood cholesterol level. One chart will give you your personal "SF1" number—this represents the maximum number of grams of saturated fat that a person of your age, sex, and activity level should eat each day to lower your cholesterol level. Your SF1 number (the letters stand for "saturated fat" this time) is the target you will use for daily saturated-fat consumption, and it equals approximately 10 percent of the total amount of calories you should consume. Once you know your SF1 number, you can then use the SF1 Food Lists to choose your foods and determine the quantities you should eat.

Using your SF1 number and the SF1 Food Lists eliminates the need for a rigid diet. There are no compulsory foods in this program and no foods you must avoid. Once you know your number, you can select any food from the SF1 List that helps you reach your goal. You don't have to deprive yourself of any of the foods you like to eat, although—to be honest—our system may guide you toward eating them less often or in smaller quantities. It will also show you how to select equally tasty alternatives that are lower in saturated fat.

In Chapter Nine, we will make it just as easy for you to determine the amount of soluble fiber you should eat each day, and we'll show you where to get it. You'll use another simple chart to find your personal "SF2" number—which represents the desirable number of grams of soluble fiber that a person of your age, sex, and activity level should eat each day to lower your cholesterol level. As you will see, your SF2 number (in this case the letters stand for "soluble fiber") is designed to provide you with about 6.75 grams of soluble fiber for each 1,000 calories of food you eat. That's an amount that will help most people lower their cholesterol levels significantly. Once you know your personal SF2 number, you can use the SF2 Food Lists to choose your high-fiber foods and determine how much of each you should eat.

As in the case of saturated fat, using your personal SF2 number and the SF2 Food Lists to make your food selections eliminates the need for a rigid diet or a fixed menu. You don't have to concentrate on only one or two foods to reach your SF2 goal, and you won't have to avoid any, either. Just select any food from the SF2 List that helps you reach your SF2 number, and enjoy it to your heart's content.

In Chapter Ten, we will describe some other strategies you can use to lower your blood cholesterol level or decrease your risk of coronary heart disease. These actions include decreasing the amount of cholesterol you eat each day (this is a separate issue from saturated fat), exercising regularly, and avoiding cigarettes. The more of these things you do, the healthier your cardiovascular system is likely to be.

In Chapter Eleven, there is a thirty-day diary you can use to monitor your progress. This diary will help you keep track of your daily accomplishments in meeting your SF1 and SF2 goals. You can also use it to make note of foods and strategies that work particularly well for you, and to identify problems and pitfalls that you want to avoid in the future. The diary pages also provide you with some helpful hints and information to assist you toward your goal.

The diary, incidentally, should be helpful to your physician, as well. The two of you can use it to determine exactly how little saturated fat and how much soluble fiber you consumed during the first thirty days. He or she may combine this information with the results of another blood cholesterol test to determine just how responsive your body is to the dietary approach for cholesterol reduction. That can be very important in determining whether any additional therapy, such as drugs, will be necessary.

In Chapter Twelve, we'll show you how to evaluate your progress. If your blood cholesterol test is repeated at this time, you can use the guidelines in that chapter (developed by the National Cholesterol Education Program) to determine if your cholesterol-lowering efforts have produced medically acceptable results. If you are making satisfactory progress, you'll continue on the same program that you followed for the first thirty days. If your cholesterol level does not appear to be dropping far enough, you'll find a second set of SF1 charts in Chapter Twelve that you can use to reduce your saturated fat even further—to 7 percent of your total caloric intake.

In Chapter Thirteen, you'll find information about the drugs that are available to lower blood cholesterol levels when dietary measures alone are not enough. You will learn how each drug works and why some drugs are used instead of others in selected cases. You'll also find a description of the most common side effects of each drug. Though we hope you won't need medications to get your cholesterol down to an acceptable level (most people don't), you will find this information helpful if you do.

You may wonder if the simple approach presented in this book can really work for a problem as complex as high blood cholesterol. The answer is: It does for most people, and it should work for you. Because each person is different, some individuals who use this plan may experience remarkable drops in their cholesterol levels, while others will not improve as much. The only way you can learn which group you are in is by following the plan as closely as you possibly can and comparing your blood cholesterol level after thirty days to your level before you started.

There are other benefits to be gained from this plan in addition to lowering blood cholesterol levels. If you are overweight and you achieve your daily goals for saturated fat (SF1) and soluble fiber (SF2) intake, you are likely to lose weight because most of your food choices will be low in calories, yet high in satisfying bulk. Your nutritional status is likely to be enhanced, too, since the foods that work well in the SF system tend to be relatively high in vitamin and mineral content for their caloric value.

So don't wait any longer to begin reducing your cholesterol. Turn the page, determine your SF1 and SF2 numbers, and start now to count out cholesterol.

8

♥ ♥ ♥ ♥

USING SF1

Count Down
on Saturated Fat

s you have already learned, there are several intake factors that
influence your LDL cholesterol level and, therefore, your total
blood cholesterol level. These include the total amount of fat—
especially the saturated fat—in your diet and the amount of dietary cholesterol that you consume each day. Though all are important, many
excellent studies, dating back as far as the 1960s, show that saturated fat
affects your blood cholesterol level more than any other intake factor—
even dietary cholesterol.

In Chapter Three, we described one of the most persuasive of these
reports, the Seven Countries Study. Equally impressive was a Harvard
School of Public Health study in 1965. Men (ages 38 to 57) were administered four-week diets that varied in the amount of fat and cholesterol
they contained. A total of thirty-six different test diets were evaluated,
with the proportion of fat in these diets ranging from 22 percent to 40

percent of total calories. Blood cholesterol levels responded differently to the various diets, and after a close analysis, researchers concluded that more than any other dietary component, variations in saturated fat bore most of the responsibility for those changes. In fact, saturated fats alone accounted for 72 percent of the variations in blood cholesterol levels, an effect considerably greater than that of dietary cholesterol.

That is why we will focus a great deal of our attention (and yours) on this area, and it is the reason why the National Cholesterol Education Program has recommended that less than 10 percent of your total daily calories should come from saturated fat. But as we pointed out in Chapter Seven, it takes a mathematical whiz to follow that advice. First you have to know how many calories you should be eating each day (that figure depends on your sex, weight, and activity level). Then you have to divide that number by ten (to determine the number of calories that should be saturated fat) and divide *that* result by nine (to determine the actual amount of fat—measured in grams—that you can eat). Finally, you would have to figure out how many grams of saturated fat there are in each food you eat.

That is a lot of work—enough to discourage many people from going further—so we created a simple system to take the mathematics away. All you have to do is find your personal SF1 number, using a chart in this chapter, and you will know the amount of saturated fat you can eat each day. The SF1 number represents the maximum amount of saturated fat, in grams, that a person of your sex, activity level, and desirable weight can consume each day without exceeding the 10 percent guideline. To make the last part of your task easier—picking the foods you should eat—you should refer frequently to the list of SF1 values for the foods you are most likely to encounter. Here's what to do to get started on the program now:

1. Use the charts on page 73 or 74 to find the desirable weight for your sex and height. This is the weight you should be for your height and bone structure—not necessarily how much you actually weigh. If you are overweight now, the foods you will be selecting under this program are likely to help you lose weight.

Chart 13

DESIRABLE WEIGHTS FOR MEN[1]
(AGES 25 AND OVER)

Height[2] Feet Inches		Small Frame	Medium Frame	Large Frame
5	2	128–134	131–141	138–150
5	3	130–136	133–143	140–153
5	4	132–138	135–145	142–156
5	5	134–140	137–148	144–160
5	6	136–142	139–151	146–164
5	7	138–145	142–154	149–168
5	8	140–148	145–157	152–172
5	9	142–151	148–160	155–176
5	10	144–154	151–163	158–180
5	11	146–157	154–166	161–184
6	0	149–160	157–170	164–188
6	1	152–164	160–174	168–192
6	2	155–168	164–178	172–197
6	3	158–172	167–182	176–202
6	4	162–176	171–187	181–207

To determine your ideal weight, find your height in the left-hand column. Then move across the page to the body frame that best describes you. For the purposes of this table, your body frame is "small" if you can wrap your left thumb and middle finger around your right wrist and have these two digits overlap. If the thumb and finger barely touch, then you have a "medium" body frame. If they don't touch at all, you have a "large" build.

[1]Weight in pounds according to frame (in indoor clothing weighing 5 lbs. for men and 3 lbs. for women).
[2]With 1-inch heel shoes on.

SOURCE OF BASIC DATA: *1979 Build Study, Society of Actuaries and Association of Life Insurance Medical Directors of America, 1980.*

Chart 13

DESIRABLE WEIGHTS FOR WOMEN[1]
(AGES 25 AND OVER)

Height[2]		Small Frame	Medium Frame	Large Frame
Feet	Inches			
4	10	102–111	109–121	118–131
4	11	103–113	111–123	120–134
5	0	104–115	113–126	122–137
5	1	106–118	115–129	125–140
5	2	108–121	118–132	128–143
5	3	111–124	121–135	131–147
5	4	114–127	124–138	134–151
5	5	117–130	127–141	137–155
5	6	120–133	130–144	140–159
5	7	123–136	133–147	143–163
5	8	126–139	136–150	146–167
5	9	129–142	139–153	149–170
5	10	132–145	142–156	152–173
5	11	135–148	145–159	155–176
6	0	138–151	148–162	158–179

To determine your ideal weight, find your height in the left-hand column. Then move across the page to the body frame that best describes you. For the purposes of this table, your body frame is "small" if you can wrap your left thumb and middle finger around your right wrist and have these two digits overlap. If the thumb and finger barely touch, then you have a "medium" body frame. If they don't touch at all, you have a "large" build.

[1]Weight in pounds according to frame (in indoor clothing weighing 5 lbs. for men and 3 lbs. for women).
[2]With 1-inch heel shoes on.

SOURCE OF BASIC DATA: *1979 Build Study, Society of Actuaries and Association of Life Insurance Medical Directors of America, 1980.*

2. Next, determine your general physical activity level:

- *Inactive:* You fall into this category if your physical activity is limited. Perhaps you do some occasional slow walking. Or you may concentrate on recreational activities such as fishing, golf (with the help of a golf cart), bowling, or horseback riding.

- *Moderately Active:* In this category, your activities would include ten to twenty minutes a day of continuous, vigorous exercise, three or more times a week. These activities could range from jogging to swimming to skiing to doubles tennis.

- *Active:* You belong in this category if you spend over twenty minutes exercising continuously and vigorously, three or more times a week. These activities might include jogging, swimming, singles tennis, or full court basketball.

3. Finally, with your ideal weight and activity level in mind, consult the chart on page 76 (men) or page 77 (women) to determine your SF1 number. You will use this number throughout the program to help you channel your eating behavior in a more positive direction. Follow the instructions that appear beneath the chart.

You will use your SF1 number to guide you in your food selections and meal planning. If you can keep your intake of saturated fats consistently *below* your SF1 number, you should be on your way toward a lower blood cholesterol level. To make your food selection easier, you will find the SF1 values for common foods in the Food Lists beginning on page 77. These lists categorize the most common sources of saturated fat in the American diet by food type (meats, dairy products, etc.). Beside each item you'll find a typical serving size, and the SF1 number for that portion of food. These numbers represent the approximate number of grams of saturated fat in the designated serving. This makes it possible to tell at a glance what you should eat to stay under your personal SF1 quota for the day. To repeat: The sum of the SF1 numbers for the foods you eat each day should not exceed your personal SF1 number.

Chart 14

PERSONAL SF1 NUMBERS: MEN

Desirable Weight	Activity Level		
	Inactive	Moderately Active	Very Active
90	14	15	16
100	16	17	18
110	17	18	20
120	19	20	21
130	20	22	23
140	22	23	25
150	23	25	27
160	25	27	28
170	26	28	30
180	28	30	32
190	30	32	34
200	31	33	36
210	33	35	37
220	34	37	39

Find the figure in the lefthand column that most closely corresponds to the desirable weight you identified in Step 1. Then move across the chart to the vertical column that corresponds to your physical activity level. At the point where your ideal weight and activity level intersect, you will find *your* personal SF1 number. This number represents the maximum amount of saturated fat (in grams) that you should consume each day.

Although there are no forbidden foods in this program, on those occasions when you do select an item such as a juicy red steak or ice cream, you can compensate by passing up other items that are high in saturated fat. *You* will be in control, because *you* will be making all the choices. And the SF1 system will take the work out of making those selections. You can have all the foods you want until the sum of their SF1 values reaches the level of your personal SF1 number. The system may sound simple, but by keeping the amount of saturated fat you eat to a particular level each day, it can have a very significant effect on your blood cholesterol level.

Chart 14

PERSONAL SF1 NUMBERS: WOMEN

Desirable Weight	Activity Level		
	Inactive	Moderately Active	Very Active
90	13	14	14
100	14	15	16
110	15	17	18
120	17	18	19
130	18	20	21
140	20	21	22
150	21	23	24
160	22	24	26
170	24	26	27
180	25	27	29
190	27	29	30
200	28	30	32
210	29	32	34
220	31	33	35

Find the figure in the lefthand column that most closely corresponds to the desirable weight you identified in Step 1. Then move across the chart to the vertical column that corresponds to your physical activity level. At the point where your ideal weight and activity level intersect, you will find *your* personal SF1 number. This number represents the maximum amount of saturated fat (in grams) that you should consume each day.

Chart 15

SF1 VALUES OF FOODS

The following tables list the SF1 values for commonly used foods. The SF1 value listed here is approximately equal to the number of grams of saturated fat in the portion. If your portion is larger or smaller, you will have to multiply or divide the SF1 value accordingly. These SF1 values have been rounded off to the nearest one-half gram, except when the amount of saturated fat in a portion is less than one-half gram, in which case the value is reported to the nearest tenth of a gram. While these values are estimates, they are accurate enough to help you choose foods low in saturated fat.

The more foods you choose from the top of each table, and the less you eat of foods at the bottom, the more your blood cholesterol level is likely to drop.

MEATS

Food	Portion	SF1
Ham slices, lean	2 slices	1.0
Kidneys, simmered	3.5 oz	1.0
Liver, braised	3.5 oz	2.0
Round, beef, lean	3.5 oz	3.0
Leg of lamb, lean	3.5 oz	3.0
Sausage, pork	2 links	3.0
Sirloin, lean	3.5 oz	3.5
Tenderloin, lean	3.5 oz	3.5
Salami, beef	2 slices	4.0
Smoked ham	3.5 oz	4.0
T-bone, lean	3.5 oz	4.0
Lamb chop, lean	3.5 oz	5.0
Veal cutlet, medium fat	3.5 oz	5.0
Corned beef	3.5 oz	6.5
Ground beef, lean	3.5 oz	7.0
Ribs, lean	3.5 oz	7.0
Sausage, beef	2 links	11.5
Bologna, beef	3-4 slices	12.0
Frankfurter, beef	2 franks	12.0
Spare ribs, pork	3.5 oz	12.0
Bacon, fried	3.5 oz	17.5

POULTRY

Food	Portion	SF1
Turkey, white meat, no skin	3.5 oz	0.4
Chicken, white meat, no skin	3.5 oz	1.0
Turkey roll	3 slices	1.5
Turkey, dark meat, no skin	3.5 oz	1.5
Chicken, dark meat, no skin	3.5 oz	2.5
Duck, no skin	3.5 oz	4.0
Bologna, turkey	3 slices	4.0
Frankfurter, chicken	2 franks	5.0
Frankfurter, turkey	2 franks	5.5

SEAFOOD

Food	Portion	SF1
Lobster	3.5 oz	0.1
Perch	3.5 oz	0.2

Food	Portion	SF1
Cod	3.5 oz	0.2
Clams	3.5 oz	0.2
Crab	3.5 oz	0.2
Pollock	3.5 oz	0.2
Haddock	3.5 oz	0.2
Shrimp	3.5 oz	0.3
Grouper	3.5 oz	0.3
Halibut	3.5 oz	0.4
Snapper	3.5 oz	0.4
Rockfish	3.5 oz	0.5
Sea bass	3.5 oz	0.5
Mussels	3.5 oz	1.0
Trout	3.5 oz	1.0
Oysters	3.5 oz	1.5
Swordfish	3.5 oz	1.5
Tuna, albacore, canned, water-pack	3.5 oz	1.5
Tuna, bluefin	3.5 oz	1.5
Salmon	3.5 oz	2.0
Anchovies, canned, in oil	5 anchovies	0.4
Herring	3.5 oz	2.5
Eel	3.5 oz	3.0
Mackerel	3.5 oz	4.0
Pompano	3.5 oz	4.5

DAIRY PRODUCTS

Food	Portion	SF1
Egg, white	1	0.0
Yogurt, plain, nonfat	8 oz.	0.2
Skim milk	8 oz.	0.3
Cottage cheese, 1% fat	4 oz.	0.5
Parmesan cheese, grated	1 tbsp.	1.0
Buttermilk	8 oz.	1.5
Egg, whole	1	1.5
Low-fat milk, 1% fat	8 oz.	1.5
Yogurt, flavored, low-fat	8 oz.	2.0
Cottage cheese, creamed	4 oz.	3.0
Low-fat milk, 2% fat	8 oz.	3.0
Mozzarella, part-skim	1 oz.	3.0
American processed cheese spread	1 oz.	4.0
American processed cheese slices	1 oz. (1.5 slices)	4.5
Cheese, whole-milk	1 oz.	5.0
Whole milk, 3.3% fat	8 oz.	5.0

Food	Portion	SF1
Yogurt, plain, whole milk	8 oz.	5.0
Ricotta, part-skim	4 oz.	5.5
Cream cheese	1 oz.	6.0
Butter	1 tbsp.	7.5
Ricotta, whole-milk	4 oz.	9.5
Quiche	⅛ of 8" diameter	23.0

GRAINS, PASTA, RICE, AND PIZZA

Food	Portion	SF1
Barley, pearled	2 tbsp.	0.0
Spaghetti, cooked	1 cup	0.1
Macaroni, cooked	1 cup	0.1
Rice, white, instant, cooked	1 cup	0.1
Cornmeal, degermed	1 cup	0.2
Flour, all-purpose or whole wheat	1 cup	0.3
Flour, wheat, cake	1 cup	0.3
Rice, brown, cooked	1 cup	0.3
Bulgur wheat, cooked	1 cup	0.5
Egg noodles, cooked	1 cup	0.5
Noodles, chow mein	1 cup	2.0
Pizza, cheese	⅛ of 15" pie	1.5

SOUPS

Food	Portion	SF1
Gazpacho	1 cup	0.3
Onion, made with water	1 cup	0.3
Beef bouillon, canned	1 cup	0.3
Black bean, canned, made with water	1 cup	0.4
Chicken broth, canned, made with water	1 cup	0.4
Tomato, made with water	1 cup	0.4
Vegetable	1 cup	0.5
Split pea with ham	1 cup	1.5
Minestrone	1 cup	1.5
Chicken noodle, canned, made with water	1 cup	1.5
Clam chowder, Manhattan style	1 cup	2.0
Chicken, chunky, canned	1 cup	2.0
Cream of chicken, canned, made with water	1 cup	2.0
Cream of mushroom, canned, made with water	1 cup	2.5
Beef, chunky, canned	1 cup	2.5
Clam chowder, New England style, with skim milk	1 cup	3.0

Food	Portion	SF1
Tomato, made with skim milk	1 cup	3.0
Cream of chicken, canned, made with skim milk	1 cup	4.5
Cream of mushroom, made with skim milk	1 cup	5.0

BREADS AND CRACKERS

Food	Portion	SF1
Melba toast, plain	1 piece	0.1
Pita bread, white	½ large shell	0.1
Tortilla, corn	1 tortilla	0.1
Saltines	1 cracker	0.1
Oat bran bread	1 slice	0.2
Bagel, plain	1, 3.5" diameter	0.3
English muffin	1 muffin	0.3
White bread, enriched	1 slice	0.3
Whole wheat bread	1 slice	0.4
Frankfurter bun	1 bun	0.5
Graham crackers	2 squares	0.5
Hamburger bun	1 bun	0.5
Pancakes, made with skim milk	1, 4" diameter	0.5
Oat bran and raisin muffin, our recipe	1 muffin	1.0
Whole wheat crackers	5 crackers	1.0
Bran muffin	1, 2.5" diameter	1.5
Corn muffin	1, 2.5" diameter	1.5
Waffle, plain, dry mix, complete	1 waffle	1.7
Doughnut, plain	1, 3.25" diameter	3.0
Croissant	1, 4.5" x 4"	3.5

CEREALS

It is impossible to list SF1 values for all brands of cereal. Use the amount of fat indicated on the package label as a general guide. Avoid cereals made with coconut, palm, or palm kernel oil, or eat them sparingly.

Food	Portion	SF1
Corn flakes	1 cup	0.0
Wheat cereal, cooked	1 cup	0.0
Wheat flakes	1 cup	0.1
40% bran flakes	1 cup	0.2
High-fiber bran cereal	1 cup	0.2
Shredded wheat squares	1 cup	0.2
Toasted oats	1 cup	0.2
Oat bran cereal	1 cup	1.0

Food	Portion	SF1
Oatmeal, cooked	1 cup	0.4
100% whole wheat bran	1 cup	0.5
Raisin bran	1 cup	1.0
Oat bran, dry	1 cup	1.5

BEANS AND LEGUMES

Food	Portion	SF1
Lentils, cooked	½ cup	0.0
Butter beans, cooked	½ cup	0.1
Kidney beans, cooked	½ cup	0.1
Lima beans, cooked	½ cup	0.1
Pinto beans, cooked	½ cup	0.1
Split peas, cooked	½ cup	0.1
White beans, cooked	½ cup	0.1
Black-eyed peas, cooked	½ cup	0.2
Garbanzo beans, cooked	½ cup	0.2

VEGETABLES

In their natural state, most vegetables contain extremely small quantities of saturated fat. Since the SF1 values for most of the vegetables in this table were much lower than 0.1 gram, we designated their SF1 values as zero. However, serving the vegetables with a rich sauce or frying them in oil will significantly raise the amount of saturated fat per portion. For example, compare the SF1 value for French-fried potatoes (2.5) with the SF1 value for a plain baked potato (0.1).

Food	Portion	SF1
Asparagus, cooked	½ cup	0.0
Beets, cooked	½ cup	0.0
Cabbage, cooked or raw	½ cup	0.0
Carrots, cooked or raw	½ cup	0.0
Cauliflower, cooked	½ cup	0.0
Celery, raw	½ cup	0.0
Corn, cooked	½ cup	0.0
Cucumbers, raw	½ cup	0.0
Eggplant, cooked	½ cup	0.0
Green beans, cooked or raw	½ cup	0.0
Lettuce	½ cup	0.0
Mushrooms, raw	½ cup	0.0
Onions, brown, cooked	½ cup	0.0
Pepper, cooked or raw	½ cup	0.0

Food	Portion	SF1
Tomatoes, raw	1 medium	0.0
Broccoli, cooked or raw	½ cup	0.1
Brussels sprouts, cooked or raw	½ cup	0.1
Onions, brown, raw	½ cup	0.1
Peas, cooked or raw	½ cup	0.1
Potato, with skin, baked, plain	1 medium	0.1
Sauerkraut, canned	½ cup	0.1
Spinach, cooked	½ cup	0.1
Squash, summer, cooked	½ cup	0.1
Zucchini, cooked or raw	½ cup	0.1
Squash, winter, cooked	½ cup	0.3
Olives, green	10 large	0.5
Spinach, creamed, frozen	½ cup	1.0
Green beans, frozen, cheese sauce	½ cup	2.0
Potatoes, French fries, fried in veg. oil	10 fries	2.5

FRUITS

Food	Portion	SF1
Applesauce, canned, unsweetened	½ cup	0.0
Apricots	3 apricots	0.0
Blueberries	½ cup	0.0
Boysenberries, canned, water-pack	½ cup	0.0
Dates	2 dates	0.0
Grapefruit	½ medium	0.0
Orange	1 small	0.0
Peach	1 medium	0.0
Pear	1 medium	0.0
Pineapple	½ cup	0.0
Plums	3 small	0.0
Prunes, canned	½ cup	0.0
Prunes, dried	3 prunes	0.0
Raspberries	½ cup	0.0
Raspberries, canned, water-pack	½ cup	0.0
Strawberries	½ cup	0.0
Tangerine	1 small	0.0
Apple, with skin	1 medium	0.1
Blackberries	½ cup	0.1
Cherries, sweet	10 cherries	0.1
Figs	1 medium	0.1
Grapes	12 grapes	0.1
Melon, cantaloupe, or honeydew	1 cup	0.1
Nectarine	1 small	0.1

COUNT OUT CHOLESTEROL

Food	Portion	SF1
Banana	1 medium	0.2
Raisins, seedless	½ cup	0.2
Avocado	1 medium	5.0

NUTS

Food	Portion	SF1
Almonds	21 nuts	1.5
Hazelnuts (filberts)	21 nuts	1.5
Pecans	8 nuts	1.5
Walnuts	7 nuts	1.5
Peanuts	32 nuts	2.0
Cashews	13 nuts	2.5
Coconut, dried, shredded, sweetened	2 tbsp.	3.0
Macadamia nuts	11 nuts	3.0
Peanut butter	2 tbsp.	3.0
Brazil nuts	8 nuts	4.5
Coconut meat, unsweetened	1 oz.	16.5

DESSERTS AND SNACKS

Food	Portion	SF1
Angel food cake	1/12 of 10" cake	0.0
Gelatin	½ cup	0.0
Popcorn, air-popped	1 cup	0.0
Pretzels	1 oz.	0.2
Popcorn, microwave-popped	1 cup	0.5
Popcorn, oil-popped	1 cup	0.5
Gingerbread	1/9 of 8" cake	1.0
Brownie, chocolate, with icing	1, 1.5" x 1.75"	1.5
Chocolate chips, chocolate flavored	¼ cup	1.5
Corn chips	1 oz.	1.5
Chocolate pudding, made with 2% milk	½ cup	2.0
Oatmeal cookies	4, 2.5" diameter	2.5
Sherbet, orange	1 cup	2.5
Tapioca, made with skim milk	½ cup	2.5
Potato chips	1 oz.	2.5
Pound cake	1/17 of loaf	3.0
Custard, from mix	½ cup	3.0
Devil's food cake, chocolate icing	1/16 of 9" cake	3.5
Ice milk, vanilla, hard	1 cup	3.5
Chocolate chip cookies	4, 2.25" diameter	4.0
Apple pie	1/6 of 9" pie	4.5

Food	Portion	SF1
Lemon meringue pie	⅙ of 9" pie	4.5
Milk chocolate	1 oz.	5.5
Chocolate, dark	1 oz.	6.0
Cheesecake, graham cracker crust	⅛ cake	9.0
Ice cream, vanilla, 10% fat	1 cup	9.0
Ice cream, vanilla, 16% fat	1 cup	14.5
Banana chocolate cream pie	⅙ of 9" pie	15.0

BEVERAGES

Food	Portion	SF1
Apple juice	8 oz.	0.0
Coffee, black	8 oz.	0.0
Cola, regular	12 oz.	0.0
Ginger ale	12 oz.	0.0
Lemonade, from mix	8 oz.	0.0
Orange drink	8 oz.	0.0
Tea, without milk	8 oz.	0.0
Tomato juice	8 oz.	0.0
Vegetable juice	8 oz.	0.0
Orange juice, fresh	8 oz.	0.1
Chocolate milk, 1% fat	8 oz.	1.5
Chocolate milk, whole milk	8 oz.	5.5
Hot chocolate, with whole milk	8 oz.	5.5
Chocolate shake	10 oz.	6.5
Eggnog	8 oz.	11.5

FATS AND OILS

Food	Portion	SF1
Cooking spray, cholesterol-free	2-sec. spray	0.1
Imitation mayonnaise, soybean	1 tbsp.	0.5
Canola oil	1 tbsp.	1.0
Imitation margarine, soft, tub	1 tbsp.	1.0
Safflower oil	1 tbsp.	1.0
Corn oil	1 tbsp.	1.5
Mayonnaise	1 tbsp.	1.5
Sunflower oil	1 tbsp.	1.5
Margarine, soft, tub	1 tbsp.	2.0
Olive oil	1 tbsp.	2.0
Sesame oil	1 tbsp.	2.0
Soybean oil	1 tbsp.	2.0
Peanut oil	1 tbsp.	2.5

Food	Portion	SF1
Shortening	1 tbsp.	3.0
Cottonseed oil	1 tbsp.	3.5
Lard	1 tbsp.	5.0
Palm oil	1 tbsp.	6.5
Butter	1 tbsp.	7.5
Palm kernel oil	1 tbsp.	11.0
Coconut oil	1 tbsp.	12.0

GRAVIES, SAUCES, AND DRESSINGS

Food	Portion	SF1
Sweet and sour sauce	½ cup	0.0
Au jus gravy, canned	½ cup	0.1
Salad dressing, low-calorie	1 tbsp.	0.2
Barbecue sauce	½ cup	0.3
Turkey gravy, canned	½ cup	0.5
Italian dressing	1 tbsp.	1.0
Russian dressing	1 tbsp.	1.0
Thousand Island dressing	1 tbsp.	1.0
Beef gravy, canned	½ cup	1.5
Blue cheese dressing	1 tbsp.	1.5
Chicken gravy, canned	½ cup	1.5
French dressing	1 tbsp.	1.5
Sour cream	1 tbsp.	1.5
White sauce	½ cup	3.0
Cheese sauce	½ cup	4.5
Béarnaise sauce	½ cup	21.0
Hollandaise sauce	½ cup	21.0

MISCELLANEOUS FOODS

Food	Portion	SF1
Baking powder	1 tsp.	0.0
Pancake syrup	1 oz.	0.0
Psyllium flower supplement	1 tbsp.	0.0
Spices and herbs	1 tsp.	0.1
Cocoa powder	2 tsp.	0.4
Nondairy creamer, powdered	1 tsp.	0.5
Tofu	5.5 oz.	0.5
Whipped topping, frozen	1 tbsp.	1.0
Half-and-half creamer	1 tbsp.	1.0
Baking chocolate	1 oz.	9.5

To give you an idea of how the SF1 system works, we've assembled three sample meal plans.

Meal Plan 1: First let's look at a *poor* example of food selection. Not everyone is conscientious about what he or she eats. Let's take the case of a 190-pound, inactive male whose ideal weight is 160. His SF1 number is 25, but with this diet he will find it impossible to stay below it:

	SF1 Value
Breakfast	
Eggs, soft-boiled (2)	3.0
Bacon, fried (3.5 oz.)	17.5
Whole wheat toast (2 slices)	0.8
with butter (1 tbsp.)	7.5
Coffee (2 cups)	0.0
with half-and-half creamer (1 tbsp.)	1.0
Lunch	
Bologna and cheese sandwich:	
Bologna (3 slices)	12.0
Whole-milk ricotta cheese (2 oz.)	4.8
Whole wheat bread (2 slices)	0.8
Lettuce	0.0
Mayonnaise (1 tsp.)	1.5
Potato chips (2 oz.)	5.0
Iced tea (8 oz.)	0.0
with sugar (2 tsp.)	0.0
Dinner	
Tossed salad: Lettuce (1 cup)	0.0
Tomato, onions	0.1
Pork spare ribs (7 oz.)	24.0
Baked potato (1)	0.1
with butter (1 tbsp.)	7.5
with sour cream (5 tbsp.)	7.5
Cooked vegetables (carrots, peas; 1 cup)	0.1
with butter (1 tbsp.)	7.5
Coffee (1 cup)	0.0
with half-and-half creamer (1 tbsp.)	1.0
Snacks, Desserts	
Lemon meringue pie (⅙ of 9" pie)	4.5
Cola drink	0.0
Total SF1 value for the day	106.2

This man's SF1 total was unacceptably high—over four times his personal SF1 number of 25.

Meal Plan 2: Now let's look at the same individual as he conscientiously uses the SF1 lists to guide his food selections. Again, based on his weight and activity level, his SF1 number is 25. Here is what his meals might look like:

	SF1 Value
Breakfast	
Oat bran cereal (1 cup)	1.0
Skim milk (8 oz.)	0.3
Grapefruit (½ medium)	0.0
Orange juice, fresh (8 oz.)	0.1
Oat bran and raisin muffin (1)	1.0
Coffee, decaf (1 cup)	0.0
Lunch	
Hamburger, lean (7 oz.) with bun, lettuce, tomato slice	14.5
with mayonnaise, imitation, soybean (1 tbsp.)	0.5
Split peas, cooked (½ cup)	0.1
Skim milk (8 oz.)	0.3
Pear (1 medium)	0.0
Iced tea	0.0
Dinner	
Halibut, broiled (7 oz.)	0.8
with lemon	0.0
Broccoli (½ cup)	0.1
Corn (½ cup)	0.0
Skim milk (8 oz.)	0.3
Snacks, Desserts	
Figs (5)	0.5
Cottage cheese, 1% fat (4 oz.)	0.5
Oat bran and raisin muffin (1)	1.0
Total SF1 value for the day	21.0

This man was able to eat his favorite foods (hamburger and halibut) in large portions and still come in well under his SF1 number of 25.

Meal Plan 3: These meals are appropriate for a moderately active 128-pound woman whose ideal weight is 120 pounds. As the chart on page 77 indicates, this woman's ideal weight and activity level give her an SF1 number of 18. That translates to a saturated-fat intake goal of less than 18 grams per day. Here is what she might consume on an average day to reach that objective:

	SF1 Value
Breakfast	
Oat bran cereal (½ cup)	0.5
with sliced banana (½ medium)	0.1
Skim milk (8 oz.)	0.3
Oat bran and raisin muffin (1)	1.0
Orange juice, fresh (8 oz.)	0.1
Coffee (1 cup)	0.0
with skim milk (1 oz.)	0.0
Lunch	
Soup, minestrone (1 cup)	1.5
Green salad (lettuce, chopped vegetables)	0.0
with Italian dressing (1 tbsp.)	1.0
Oat bran and raisin muffin (1)	1.0
Skim milk (8 oz.)	0.3
Dinner	
Chicken, light meat, no skin (3.5 oz.)	1.0
Steamed vegetables (1 cup: carrots, green beans)	0.0
Kidney beans (½ cup, cooked)	0.1
Coffee (1 cup)	0.0
with skim milk (1 oz.)	0.0
Snacks, Desserts	
Apple pie (1 slice)	4.5
Popcorn, air-popped (1 cup)	0.0
Total SF1 value for the day	11.4

This woman was able to eat three full meals and several tasty snacks, and still stay well under her SF1 number of 18.

In the last two examples, the nutritious and interesting menus show that you don't have to sacrifice the pleasures of eating to stay under your SF1 number. As well as cutting down on your blood cholesterol level, there are other benefits to eating this way. In the second example, this overweight man ate quite well but also consumed fewer calories than he once did. Consistently eating this way will enable him to reach his ideal weight. (Becoming more active physically wouldn't hurt, either.)

Now that you know your personal SF1 number, take a few minutes to scan the SF1 Food Lists to see what your own daily diet can look like. After a few days, you won't need to refer to the lists very often. You will become so familiar with the SF1 values of the foods you eat that your meal-planning decisions will become almost automatic. But until then, the lists will help you recognize those foods that contribute large amounts of saturated fat to your diet. These are the foods that you should eat in smaller amounts or choose less often than in the past.

The material that follows discusses some of the food groups that create problems for people who must limit their intake of saturated fat. In it, you'll find helpful hints from the National Cholesterol Education Program and other reliable sources on how to deal with these foods without giving them up completely.

MEATS

Meats have been the primary target of many cholesterol-lowering programs because they generally contain significant amounts of saturated fat and cholesterol. But it is not necessary to give up meat entirely to meet the goals of this program and stay under your personal SF1 number. The trick is to select the right cuts of meat, control the size of the portions you eat, and use cooking techniques that minimize the amount of fat that actually reaches your plate.

Though some cuts of meat are truly loaded with saturated fat, many others contain fairly modest amounts and can be eaten with reasonable frequency. In general, you should select cuts without visible fat or marbling, and trim off as much as you can of the fat that is present. The following cuts are examples of the leanest:

Beef	Veal	Pork	Lamb
Round	All trimmed	Tenderloin	Leg
Sirloin	cuts except	Leg (fresh)	Arm
Chuck	commercially	Shoulder	Loin
Loin	ground	(arm or picnic)	

Select "good" grades of meat rather than "choice" or "prime." The "good" grade is lower in fat than the others but is still tasty and high in protein and iron. Be cautious about buying meats that are labeled "light," "lite," "leaner," or "lower fat," because these selections may still be high in saturated fat. Read the label for precise information about the grams of fat per serving or slice, or the exact percentage of fat that is present.

Also cut down the amount of bacon and processed meats such as bologna, salami, hot dogs, and sausage made of beef or pork. These meats may contain as much as 60 to 80 percent of their calories in the form of fat, much of it saturated. Most people find the low-fat alternatives made from turkey (check the amount of fat on the label, because there are high-fat turkey products, too) are just as satisfying to their taste. Although organ meats such as liver, sweetbreads, and kidneys are relatively low in saturated fat, they are quite high in cholesterol (see Chapter Ten), so their intake should be limited also.

The way you prepare your meats can have a significant effect on how much saturated fat you end up eating. You can lower that figure by broiling, baking, or roasting meats on a rack that allows the fat to drip away. If you wish to pan-fry or sauté meats, use a nonstick cooking pan or a cholesterol-free cooking spray instead of butter, lard, margarine, or oil. (Margarines and oils do contain saturated fats—in some cases, large quantities.) You can also decrease the amount of saturated fat in each portion of meat you serve by "extending" your meat dishes with beans, vegetables, pasta, grains, or other foods that are naturally low in fat. Don't spoil any of these cooking efforts by serving your meat with sauces that are high in fat.

POULTRY

Ounce for ounce, the poultry group tends to be lower in saturated fat than the meat group, yet it is high in protein and makes any meal feel substantial. You should be aware that light meat contains significantly less saturated fat and cholesterol than dark meat. Also, goose and duck—though members of the poultry group—are not low in these substances. Chart 16 gives information you can use when selecting poultry at the market or when eating out. You will find much more in the SF1 Food Lists on pages 78–86.

As you can see above, the amount of saturated fat and cholesterol in poultry can be significantly reduced if you remove the skin before you cook it. Baking and broiling are preferable to deep frying.

SEAFOOD

Most fish are lower in saturated fat and cholesterol than meat and poultry. By eating fish two or three times a week in place of meat or poultry, you may significantly lower your intake of saturated fat. You'll find particularly low amounts of saturated fat in fish such as halibut, cod, sea bass, whitefish, rockfish, snapper, haddock, and perch. Shellfish that are sedentary (clams, scallops, mussels) are very low in saturated fat and moderately low in cholesterol. Shrimp, though low in saturated fat, is quite high in cholesterol (195 mg per 3 1/2 oz. portion). Eel is also high in cholesterol (161 mg).

You need to be careful not to undermine the excellent cholesterol-lowering properties of seafood by adding saturated fat to your dishes when you cook and serve them. Broiling, baking, and poaching are much preferred to deep frying. If you pan-fry or sauté your fish, use cooking spray or polyunsaturated oils, not butter, or try a nonstick pan. When you are serving, substitute a twist of lemon for rich sauces.

MILK

Milk is a tasty and nutritious food that provides abundant quantities of protein and several essential vitamins and minerals. It comes in several different forms: whole milk (3.3 percent fat), low-fat (2 percent or 1 percent fat), and nonfat or skim (virtually free of fat). Depending on which type you drink, milk can be either an aid to your cholesterol-lowering program or a factor that interferes with the attainment of your goal. You

Chart 16

**FAT AND CHOLESTEROL CONTENT OF
SELECTED CUTS OF POULTRY**

Cut (3½ oz., cooked)	Total Fat (grams)	Saturated Fat (grams)	Cholesterol (milligrams)
Turkey, white meat without skin	1.9	0.4	86
Turkey, white meat with skin	4.6	1.3	95
Turkey, dark meat without skin	4.3	1.4	112
Turkey, dark meat with skin	7.1	2.1	117
Chicken, white meat without skin	4.1	1.1	75
Chicken, white meat with skin	10.9	3.0	84
Chicken, dark meat without skin	9.7	2.7	93
Chicken, dark meat with skin	15.8	4.4	91
Duck, flesh only	11.2	4.2	89

can keep all of the nutrition and avoid all of the cholesterol-raising elements simply by switching to nonfat milk. Although almost all of the fat is gone, this product contains essentially the same amount of minerals, vitamins, protein, and calcium as whole milk.

At first glance, 2 percent or even 3.3 percent fat content doesn't seem like much, but that figure is based on weight—including the weight of the water in the milk. If you consider only the substances in milk that contain calories, the fat in whole milk accounts for 74 of the 150 calories in each cup. That means that whole milk is really *49 percent fat*—much too high for any cholesterol-lowering program, particularly since most of this fat (62 percent of it) is saturated. Though switching to low-fat (2 per-

CAN CALCIUM LOWER YOUR CHOLESTEROL?

Calcium may do more than protect you against osteoporosis. Several studies have found that the consumption of calcium might reduce blood cholesterol levels, too. In 1992, researchers at the University of Minnesota and Hennepin County Medical Center reported giving calcium carbonate (the equivalent of a Tums tablet three times a day) to patients with mild to moderate elevations of cholesterol, while also placing them on a low-fat, low-cholesterol diet that began eight weeks before administration of the calcium. After six weeks on the calcium supplements, patients experienced a 4 percent reduction in their LDL cholesterol, and a 4 percent increase in their HDL cholesterol, that could be attributed to calcium.

More studies need to be conducted. In the meantime, calcium supplements make most sense for osteoporosis prevention, with a potential for modestly reducing your blood cholesterol levels, too.

cent) milk helps, it doesn't solve the problem. Of the 121 calories in a cup of low-fat milk, 42 are in the form of fat (mostly saturated), which means that 35 percent of the calories are coming from fat. By contrast, only 5 percent of the calories in nonfat milk comes from fat. Clearly, nonfat milk is your best choice.

Some people have difficulty making the transition from whole to nonfat milk. They've become so accustomed to the rich taste of whole milk that nonfat seems flavorless by comparison and hard for them to drink. If that's your experience, make the transition gradually, one step at a time. Switch first to 2 percent milk for a few weeks and then to 1 percent for a few more weeks. Finally, take the next—and permanent—step to nonfat. You'll get used to it more quickly than you might think, and if you are like most people, you will have trouble returning to the fattier versions.

SELECTING CHEESE CAUTIOUSLY

Like milk, cheese is an excellent source of protein. That's why many people use cheese as a meat substitute when trying to lower their cholesterol. This is a serious mistake, as ounce for ounce almost all cheeses are just as high in cholesterol as meats and poultry, but much higher in saturated fat. The following comparison provided by the National Cholesterol Education Program tells the story clearly.

Fat—mostly saturated fat—makes up 65 to 75 percent of the calories found in most cheeses, so it is essential that you control the amount you eat, either by eating cheese less frequently or by eating smaller portions. It doesn't take much cheese to put you over your SF1 quota for the day. Two slices of American cheese, for instance, contain as much saturated fat as about three one-teaspoon pats of butter. Similar amounts of fat are contained in most cheeses, including Brie, provolone, Romano, Gouda, Swiss, Edam, brick, blue, Gruyere, Muenster, Parmesan, Jack, Roquefort, Cheddar, and cream cheese. Whole-milk ricotta contains almost twice as much fat.

In many supermarkets, you will find so-called "low-fat" alternatives to the standard cheeses—for example, many stores now carry "low-fat" or "part-skim" varieties of cheeses such as mozzarella and ricotta. But though these cheeses have less fat than their whole-milk relatives, they are by no means low in fat. Part-skim mozzarella has almost 3 grams of saturated fat per ounce. That's about what you will find in a 3 1/2-ounce portion of round steak, and more than twice as much as in a 3 1/2-ounce portion of skinless chicken (white meat).

So don't be fooled by the enticing names attached to cheese products. Read the label for the exact amount of fat (in grams) contained in each ounce of cheese or in each portion (make sure you know the size of the portion, too). That is the only way you can tell if that particular cheese is a good one for your cholesterol-lowering needs.

Chart 17			
POULTRY, MEAT, AND CHEESE: A COMPARISON			
Product (3 oz.)	Total Fat (grams)	Saturated Fat (grams)	Cholesterol (milligrams)
Beef, top round	6	2	84
Chicken, broiler/fryer without skin, white meat	5	1	85
Low-fat cottage cheese (1% fat)	1	1	4
Part-skim mozzarella	14	9	48
Mozzarella	18	11	66
Natural cheddar	28	18	90
Cream cheese	30	19	93

By the way, you don't have to give up your favorite cheeses forever to keep your cholesterol down. But you may have to eat them less often and in smaller portions. You should also try tasting some of the cheeses that are lower in saturated fat. One of the best choices in this category is low-fat (1 percent fat) cottage cheese (only 0.7 grams of saturated fat in a 4-ounce portion). Some people also enjoy tofu (soybean curd), which—though not a cheese—is similar in texture to cheese curd and quite low in fat.

ICE CREAM

It is almost un-American to suggest giving up ice cream, so we won't do that. But you should be aware that just one cup of rich vanilla ice cream contains about 15 grams of saturated fat and 90 milligrams of cholesterol. For many people, that single cup wipes out a good share of the SF1 points for the day and delivers about one-third of the maximum amount of cholesterol that should prudently be consumed. So don't eat this popular dish too often, and when you do, keep your portion small. Whenever you can, substitute sherbet or ice milk; that will cut your saturated-fat intake by about 80 percent and your cholesterol consumption by about 85 percent. Better yet, switch to nonfat frozen yogurt and you'll nearly eliminate the saturated fat and cholesterol.

MAKING WISE SUBSTITUTIONS

You've already seen how the substitution of one tasty food for another can dramatically reduce the amount of saturated fat you'll consume. But it's not always easy to know which substitutions are really going to do the job for you. A simple rule to follow is to seek out the foods that are at the top of each SF1 Food List category and substitute them as often as possible for foods at the bottom of that category. The more substitutions you make, the lower your saturated-fat intake will be, and the more likely you are to lower your blood cholesterol level.

Another helpful rule is to seek out foods that are high in complex carbohydrates and use them as often as possible. These foods include vegetables, fruits, rice, pasta, dried beans, and potatoes. These basic foods are almost always very low in saturated fat, yet they are rich in essential vitamins and minerals. They are also a valuable source of soluble fiber, which is an important part of this cholesterol-lowering program. So make sure that your shopping cart and your plate are filled with complex-carbohydrate foods. That is one of the best ways to avoid exceeding your SF1 quota each day and to count out cholesterol.

LOW-SATURATED-FAT MAIN DISHES

As you will learn throughout Chapter Eleven, there are many substitutions of ingredients you can make in your favorite recipes to adapt them for lower-saturated-fat dining. In the meantime, to get you off on the right foot, we asked the Good Housekeeping Institute to create some tempting main dishes that are low in saturated fat. Give them a try. They are delicious and healthy, and you will probably decide to prepare them again and again.

Broiled Salmon Steaks with Parsley Sauce

1 medium-sized lemon
4 small salmon steaks, each 3/4" thick
salt (optional)
pepper vegetable cooking spray
1 cup packed chopped parsley
1 chicken-flavor bouillon cube or envelope*
1 tablespoon margarine

*Use low-salt bouillon, if desired.

1. About 25 minutes before serving, preheat broiler if manufacturer directs. Cut 4 thin slices from lemon; set aside for garnish. From remaining lemon, squeeze 1 tablespoon juice; set aside.
2. Sprinkle salmon steaks lightly with salt and pepper. Lightly spray rack in broiling pan with vegetable cooking spray. Place salmon steaks on rack; broil about 10 minutes, or until fish flakes easily when tested with a fork, turning once with pancake turner.
3. Meanwhile, in blender at medium speed, blend parsley, bouillon, margarine, 1/3 cup water, and reserved lemon juice until smooth, stopping

occasionally to scrape blender with rubber spatula. In 1-quart saucepan over high heat, heat parsley mixture to boiling, stirring occasionally.

4. To serve, place a salmon steak on each of four dinner plates. Spoon some parsley sauce around each salmon steak. Garnish with lemon slice.

Makes 4 servings. About 275 calories, 94 mg cholesterol per serving. SF1 value: 2.0; SF2 value: 0.4.

Skillet Chicken with Vegetables

2 whole medium-sized chicken breasts
1 tablespoon olive oil
1 pound unpeeled sweet potatoes, cut into 1" slices
1 cup apple juice
1 teaspoon salt-free herb and spice seasoning
1/2 medium-sized bunch broccoli, cut into 2" by 1/2" pieces
1 tablespoon cornstarch

1. About 1 hour before serving, remove skin, excess fat, and bones from chicken breasts; cut chicken into bite-sized chunks.

2. In 12" skillet over medium heat, in hot olive oil, cook chicken until lightly browned on all sides, stirring often.

3. Add sweet potatoes, apple juice, and salt-free herb and spice seasoning; heat to boiling. Reduce heat to low; cover and simmer 15 minutes. Add broccoli, and continue cooking about 15 minutes longer, or until chicken and vegetables are tender.

4. In cup, stir cornstarch and 2 tablespoons water until smooth; gradually stir into hot liquid in skillet, stirring constantly until mixture thickens slightly and boils.

Makes 4 servings. About 360 calories, 73 mg cholesterol per serving. SF1 value: 1.5; SF2 value: 2.5.

Linguine Misto

6 medium-sized carrots
1 16-ounce package linguine
2 tablespoons olive oil
2 large garlic cloves, minced
12 ounces mushrooms, sliced
2 medium-sized onions, thinly sliced
2 medium-sized celery stalks, thinly sliced
1/4 cup lemon juice
1 tablespoon oregano leaves
1/2 teaspoon pepper
1 tablespoon cornstarch

1. About 1 1/2 hours before serving, cut each carrot lengthwise into thin slices; then cut slices into linguine-thin strips.

2. Prepare linguine as label directs; drain; keep warm.

3. Meanwhile, in 6-quart saucepot over medium heat, in hot olive oil, cook carrots, garlic, and remaining ingredients, except cornstarch, 5 minutes, stirring often. Add 1 cup water; heat to boiling; reduce heat to low, cover, and simmer about 10 minutes, or until carrots are tender-crisp.

4. In cup, stir cornstarch and 2 tablespoons water until smooth; gradually stir into hot liquid in saucepot and cook, stirring constantly, until mixture thickens slightly and boils.

5. Add linguine to carrot mixture; toss.

Makes 6 servings. About 385 calories, 0 mg cholesterol per serving. SF1 value: 1.0; SF2 value: 3.0.

9

♥ ♥ ♥ ♥

USING SF2
Count Up on Soluble Fiber

I n the last chapter, you learned how to control intake factors by focusing on saturated fat. Now you will see how the same kind of attention—this time to soluble fiber, an absorption factor—will help you by blocking the body's reabsorption from the intestines of substances that your liver uses to manufacture cholesterol. Instead of entering the bloodstream, these substances become bound to the fiber, which then carries them out of the body in the stool. This deprives the liver of the materials it needs to manufacture cholesterol, forcing it to use LDL drawn out of your bloodstream instead. That is what causes your blood cholesterol level to go down.

Soluble fiber is found in foods of plant origin. It is not the only fiber present—in fact, most foods have considerably more insoluble than soluble fiber. (The sum of the soluble and insoluble fiber is referred to as the "*total* dietary fiber" of a food.) But it is only the soluble form that has a powerful cholesterol-lowering effect. Though there are some definite benefits to eating insoluble fiber, decreasing your blood cholesterol level is not one of them.

Soluble fiber can be one of your strongest allies in the battle against high blood cholesterol. Unlike saturated fat, which you are trying to avoid, soluble fiber is something you may need to consume in larger quantity. Your personal SF2 number—which you will calculate in this chapter—will tell you just how large this quantity should be.

There are many studies providing strong evidence that soluble fiber can lower blood cholesterol levels. Much of the research was done using beans, a food rich in soluble fiber. In 1984, Dr. James W. Anderson and his colleagues at the University of Kentucky incorporated 115 grams (about 4 ounces) of dried beans each day into the daily diets of men with very high cholesterol levels (they used pinto and navy beans, served cooked or in bean soup). At the beginning of the study, these individuals had total cholesterol concentrations exceeding 260. On the bean-rich diet, their total cholesterol levels dropped 19 percent—about 55 points. Their LDL levels decreased more than their HDL levels, thus improving their TC/HDL ratio and reducing their risk of heart disease even further. There was some additional good news—these positive changes occurred rapidly. Not only did it take just twenty-one days for the 19 percent decrease to occur, but most of this decline took place within the first eleven days.

In 1985, Dr. Anderson reported the results of another study, in which supplements of canned beans (about one-half cup a day) were fed to ten men with cholesterol levels greater than 260. After three weeks on the bean diet, blood cholesterol levels fell an average of 13 percent—from 289 to 251.

Oat bran is another excellent source of soluble fiber that has been well studied. It is high in total dietary fiber, and 50 percent of that fiber is soluble. Just one-third cup of oat bran provides 4.2 grams of total fiber, with 2.0 grams in the soluble form. A series of recent studies has helped make the case for oat bran.

At the University of Kentucky, men with high cholesterol levels (over 260) were alternately put on two diets that were identical except that one included 100 grams of oat bran a day, provided in hot cereals and muffins. On this oat bran diet, the total blood cholesterol levels in the men fell an average of 13 percent after just ten days. By contrast, there were no changes in blood cholesterol levels on the diet without oat bran.

HDL levels stayed about the same on both diets. Although the study, reported in 1981, was designed for only a ten-day period for each diet, two patients did stay on the oat bran eating program for an additional four days; their total cholesterol concentrations declined an additional 8 percent between days ten and fourteen.

Another study at the University of Kentucky put a group of men with high blood cholesterol levels (over 260) on a control diet for seven days. Then for the next twenty-one days, that diet was supplemented with 100 grams a day (about 3 1/2 ounces) of oat bran, served either as a bowl of hot cereal or as five oat bran muffins. After three weeks on the oat bran diet, total cholesterol levels had fallen an average of 19 percent below their levels during the control diet. The LDL portion fell much more than the HDL portion (23 percent to 6 percent), leaving these men with a much more favorable TC/HDL ratio and a lower risk of coronary heart disease (as long as they maintained that improvement).

Ten of the men in this study did sustain these changes. They continued on a high-carbohydrate, high-fiber diet for nearly six months, incorporating either one-half cup of oat bran or one-half to one cup of cooked dried beans into their meals each day. After twenty-four weeks, total blood cholesterol levels were an average of 26 percent lower than when the study began. The investigators kept tracking four of these individuals for a total of ninety-nine weeks each; in the end, they found a 29 percent drop in LDL cholesterol, and a 9 percent *rise* in HDL cholesterol.

Still another study, reported in 1984, involved twelve healthy college students, who were asked to maintain their usual diet, except for the addition of four oat bran or wheat bran muffins per day, for a period of six weeks. Though the wheat bran muffins did not significantly influence blood cholesterol levels, the muffins made of oat bran (50 grams a day) decreased average total cholesterol levels from 184 to 164—about a 12 percent reduction.

In a study published in 1988, researchers at the University of California, Irvine, compared the effect of oat bran versus wheat bran upon total blood cholesterol values. Seventy-two medical students completed the study, in which they were divided into three groups. Some ate only oat bran muffins, others ate only wheat bran muffins, and a third group ate muffins that were a combination of oat and wheat bran. The daily dose of oat bran in the first group was quite low, equal to 17 grams, or two rounded tablespoons per day. Even so, after twenty-eight days, these individuals had experienced a 5.3 percent reduction in total cholesterol levels and an 8.7 percent reduction in LDL cholesterol values. No changes were seen in the subjects eating either the wheat or the combination muffins.

University of California researchers, analyzing the data from several studies (including their own) in which oat bran was consumed for several weeks, suggested that the following formula could be used to estimate the impact of oat bran on a person's blood cholesterol level:

0.156 x (grams oat bran/day) + 1 = percent decrease in cholesterol

Using this formula, 50 grams of oat bran per day (about 2 1/2 oat bran muffins) could produce about a 8.8 percent decline in total cholesterol. By raising the oat bran intake to 100 grams, the decrease could be even greater—16.6 percent.

Beans and Oat Bran Are Not the Only Answer

Although beans and oats deserve an important role in any cholesterol-lowering plan, there is nothing magical about either of these foods. It is the *soluble fiber* in them that causes cholesterol levels to go down, and any food (or combination of foods) that provides the same amount of soluble fiber can be expected to produce similar decreases in blood cholesterol levels. So even though eating some beans and oat bran each day will make it easier to consume the amount of soluble fiber you need, you shouldn't rely exclusively on them—or any other food—for this purpose. The more foods you use, the more interesting and nutritious your diet will be.

HOW MUCH SOLUBLE FIBER DO YOU NEED?

A formula for calculating the amount of fiber you should eat has been suggested by Dr. James Anderson and his colleagues, based on research in his own laboratory and the studies of others. His guidelines take into account the relationship between the amount of soluble fiber in the diet and blood cholesterol levels. Dr. Anderson recommends that people with high blood cholesterol eat between 6 and 7.5 grams of soluble fiber for every 1,000 calories they consume, up to a maximum daily limit of 18 grams of soluble fiber per day. This maximum is equivalent to about 50 grams of *total* dietary fiber per day. (There is a limit to the amount of fiber a person can eat, because at very high levels of fiber intake some unwanted side effects may begin to appear. See page 121.)

As helpful as Dr. Anderson's formula is, it is more accessible once all the mathematical calculations have been performed—so we have done that for you. The charts below and opposite will enable you to determine quickly the amount of soluble fiber you should consume each day—in grams. Use your ideal weight figure and activity level from Chapter Eight to find your personal SF2 number (in this case, the initials refer to "soluble fiber"). Then, later in this chapter, you'll find SF2 Food Lists

---

Chart 18

PERSONAL SF2 NUMBERS: MEN

Note: A maximum of 18 grams of soluble fiber per day is recommended

Desirable Weight	Activity Level		
	Inactive	Moderately Active	Very Active
90	9	9	10
100	9	10	11
110	10	11	12
120	11	12	13
130	12	13	14
140	13	14	15
150	14	15	16
160	15	16	17
170	16	17	18
180	17	18	18
190	18	18	18
200	18	18	18
210	18	18	18
220	18	18	18

For instructions, see chart opposite.

Chart 18

PERSONAL SF2 NUMBERS: WOMEN

Note: A maximum of 18 grams of soluble fiber per day is recommended

Desirable	Activity Level		
Weight	Inactive	Moderately Active	Very Active
90	8	8	9
100	9	9	10
110	9	10	11
120	10	11	12
130	11	12	13
140	12	13	14
150	13	14	15
160	14	15	16
170	14	15	17
180	15	16	17
190	16	17	18
200	17	18	18
210	18	18	18
220	18	18	18

Locate your ideal weight on the chart, and then your activity level, using the same values as in Chapter Eight. At the point where these columns intersect, you will find a number that represents the amount of soluble fiber (in grams) that you should eat each day. This is your SF2 number.

---

that will provide you with the SF2 values for the same foods on the SF1 list. You'll use these tables to determine what you need to eat each day to meet or exceed your SF2 quota.

If you are anything like the average American—who eats between 10 and 15 grams of *total* fiber per day—you are probably quite a bit short of your SF2 number. That's because, on average, only 30 percent of the total fiber you eat is in the soluble form. To get the amount you need, you have to pick some foods each day that are high in this remarkable substance. We will show you how to do that now.

SELECTING FOODS THAT CONTAIN SOLUBLE FIBER

The key to lowering blood cholesterol levels with dietary fiber is know-ing which foods contain large quantities of *soluble* fiber. Eating foods that are high in *total* dietary fiber is not good enough, since the proportion of fiber that is soluble varies from food to food. The following example demonstrates how one food that is higher in *total* dietary fiber may actu-ally have less *soluble* fiber than another food that is lower in *total* fiber.

Food	Total Fiber in Typical Serving: grams	Soluble: grams (% of total grams)	Insoluble: grams (% of total grams)
Graham crackers (2 squares)	2.8	0.5 (18%)	2.3 (82%)
Pinto beans (1/2 cup)	5.3	2.0 (38%)	3.3 (62%)
Oat bran (1/3 cup, dry)	4.2	2.0 (48%)	2.2 (52%)
Peach (medium size)	1.6	0.6 (38%)	1.0 (62%)

As you can see, two squares of graham crackers—though relatively high in *total* dietary fiber—actually have less *soluble* fiber than the medium-size peach. That's because 38 percent of the fiber in the peach is soluble, compared to only 18 percent of the fiber in the graham crackers.

Incidentally, until recently it was not easy to determine the amount of soluble fiber in various foods. The measurement of soluble fiber requires very complex analysis in the laboratory, and few researchers performed them. Furthermore, there has been a controversy over how these tests should be done, so findings for the same foods varied from one laboratory to another. But now there is general agreement about how these tests should be carried out and reliable figures are finally available for many, though not all, foods. Because of the expense involved, most foods have been analyzed only for their *total* dietary fiber content, so that is the value you are likely to find when you read the nutrition labels on cereal boxes and other food products. You won't find *any* figures for sol-uble fiber on the great majority of foods that contain it. Also, many of the foods rich in soluble fiber—fruits, vegetables, grains, beans, and le-gumes—don't come with nutritional labels at all, or the labels they have do not contain information about the fiber content. So how can you tell which foods to eat?

We have tried to make the job simple for you in the SF2 Food Lists, which clearly identify the approximate amount of soluble fiber in a wide variety of foods. These values correspond very closely to the grams of soluble fiber contained in typical food portions.

A quick scan of these lists will show you how many tasty foods are available to help you meet your needs for soluble fiber. You'll find some foods that are particularly high in soluble fiber, to help ensure that you will reach your SF2 goal—even on those days when you are not in the mood for a lot of food.

Chart 19

SF2 VALUES OF FOODS

The following tables list the SF2 values for commonly used foods. The SF2 value listed here is approximately equal to the number of grams of soluble fiber in the portion. If your portion is larger or smaller, you will have to multiply or divide the SF2 value accordingly. These SF2 values have been rounded off to the nearest one-half gram, except when the amount of soluble fiber in a portion is less than one-half gram, in which case the value is reported to the nearest tenth of a gram. While the SF2 values are estimates, they will guide you to make appropriate food selections to meet your soluble fiber goal.

The more foods you choose from the top of the table, the more quickly you will reach your SF2 goal for the day.

We've also listed foods that are low in soluble fiber, so you won't be lulled into thinking you have reached your goal by eating foods that don't live up to their looks.

MEATS
Meat does not contain any soluble fiber.

POULTRY
Poultry does not contain any soluble fiber.

SEAFOOD
Fish and shellfish do not contain any soluble fiber.

DAIRY PRODUCTS
Dairy products do not contain any soluble fiber.

GRAINS, PASTA, RICE, AND PIZZA

Food	Portion	SF2
Cornmeal, degermed	1 cup	4.0
Flour, all-purpose or whole wheat	1 cup	2.0
Barley, pearled	2 tbsp.	1.0
Flour, wheat, cake	1 cup	1.0
Spaghetti, cooked	1 cup	0.5
Egg noodles, cooked	1 cup	0.5
Pizza, cheese*	⅛ of 15" pie	0.0
Rice, brown, cooked	1 cup	0.4
Macaroni, cooked	1 cup	0.3
Bulgur wheat, cooked	1 cup	0.2
Rice, white, instant, cooked	1 cup	0.2
Noodles, chow mein	1 cup	0.5

*The SF2 value for pizza will be higher if the pizza is topped with a large quantity of vegetables before cooking.

SOUPS

Laboratory values for soluble fiber are not available for most of the foods in this category. In some cases, the SF2 values in this table are based on an assumption that 30 percent of the total dietary fiber is in the soluble form. The SF2 values of several foods in this table are based on typical recipes for those foods. These estimates are close enough to use for selecting foods to meet your daily goal for soluble fiber.

Food	Portion	SF2
Vegetable	1 cup	1.5
Split pea with ham	1 cup	1.5
Minestrone	1 cup	1.0
Gazpacho	1 cup	0.5
Onion, made with water	1 cup	0.5
Black bean, canned, made with water	1 cup	0.4
Clam chowder, Manhattan style	1 cup	0.4
Clam chowder, New England style, with skim milk	1 cup	0.4
Tomato, made with skim milk	1 cup	0.3
Tomato, made with water	1 cup	0.3
Beef, chunky, canned	1 cup	0.2
Cream of mushroom, canned, made with water	1 cup	0.2
Cream of mushroom, made with skim milk	1 cup	0.2
Chicken noodle, canned, made with water	1 cup	0.1
Chicken, chunky, canned	1 cup	0.1
Beef bouillon, canned	1 cup	0.0

Food	Portion	SF2
Chicken broth, canned, made with water	1 cup	0.0
Cream of chicken, canned, made with water	1 cup	0.0
Cream of chicken, canned, made with skim milk	1 cup	0.0

BREADS AND CRACKERS

The SF2 values for soluble fiber in this category are based on typical recipes for these foods. These estimates are close enough to use for selecting foods to meet your daily goal for soluble fiber.

Food	Portion	SF2
Oat bran and raisin muffin, our recipe	1 muffin	1.5
Tortilla, corn	1 tortilla	1.0
Bagel, plain	1, 3.5" diameter	0.5
Bran muffin	1, 2.5" diameter	0.5
Corn muffin	1, 2.5" diameter	0.5
English muffin	1 muffin	0.5
Frankfurter bun	1 bun	0.5
Graham crackers	2 squares	0.5
Hamburger bun	1 bun	0.5
Oat bran bread	1 slice	0.5
Pita bread	½ large shell	0.5
Waffle, plain, dry mix, complete	1 waffle	0.3
Whole wheat crackers	5 crackers	0.4
Pancakes, made with skim milk	1, 4" diameter	0.3
Saltines	1 cracker	0.0
White bread, enriched	1 slice	0.3
Whole wheat bread	1 slice	0.3
Croissant	1, 4.5" x 4"	0.2
Doughnut, plain	1, 3.25" diameter	0.2
Melba toast, plan	1 piece	0.1

CEREALS

It is impossible to list SF2 values for all brands of cereal. Use the amount of total dietary fiber indicated on the package label as a general guide. For wheat-based cereals, assume that 25 percent of the total dietary fiber is soluble; for oat-based cereals, assume that 50 percent is soluble.

Food	Portion	SF2
Oat bran, dry	1 cup	6.0
100% whole wheat bran	1 cup	5.0
High-fiber bran cereal	1 cup	5.0

Food	Portion	SF2
Oat bran cereal	1 cup	2.0
Oatmeal, cooked	1 cup	2.0
40% bran flakes	1 cup	1.0
Raisin bran	1 cup	1.0
Shredded wheat squares	1 cup	0.5
Toasted oats	1 cup	0.5
Wheat flakes	1 cup	0.5
Corn flakes	1 cup	0.2
Wheat cereal, cooked	1 cup	0.2

BEANS

Food	Portion	SF2
Black-eyed peas, cooked	½ cup	5.5
Kidney beans, cooked	½ cup	3.0
Pinto beans, cooked	½ cup	2.0
Garbanzo beans, cooked	½ cup	1.5
Split peas, cooked	½ cup	1.5
White beans, cooked	½ cup	1.5
Butter beans, cooked	½ cup	1.0
Lentils, cooked	½ cup	1 0
Lima beans, cooked	½ cup	1 0

VEGETABLES

The SF2 values for some raw vegetables differ from the SF2 values when these vegetables are cooked. This is not because the vegetables gain or lose soluble fiber in the cooking process, but because the size of vegetables may change (and therefore, the amount that will fit into a given volume).

Food	Portion	SF2
Peas, cooked	½ cup	2.0
Potato, with skin, baked, plain	1 medium	2 0
Brussels sprouts, cooked or raw	½ cup	1.5
Corn, cooked	½ cup	1.5
Zucchini, cooked	½ cup	1.5
Beets, cooked	½ cup	1.0
Broccoli, cooked or raw	½ cup	1.0
Cabbage, cooked	½ cup	1.0
Carrots, cooked	½ cup	1 0
Eggplant, cooked	½ cup	1 0
Onions, brown, cooked or raw	½ cup	1.0

Food	Portion	SF2
Peas, raw	½ cup	1.0
Sauerkraut, canned	½ cup	1.0
Zucchini, raw	½ cup	1.0
Asparagus, cooked	½ cup	0.5
Cabbage, raw	½ cup	0.5
Carrots, raw	½ cup	0.5
Cauliflower, cooked	½ cup	0.5
Green beans, cooked	½ cup	0.5
Olives, green	10 large	0.5
Spinach, cooked	½ cup	0.5
Celery, raw	½ cup	0.4
Green beans, raw	½ cup	0.4
Squash, winter, cooked	½ cup	0.4
Green beans, frozen, cheese sauce	½ cup	0.3
Mushrooms, raw	½ cup	0.3
Pepper, cooked or raw	½ cup	0.3
Spinach, creamed, frozen	½ cup	0.3
Squash, summer, cooked	½ cup	0.3
Cucumbers, raw	½ cup	0.2
Lettuce	½ cup	0.2
Potatoes, French fries, fried in veg. oil	10 fries	0.2
Tomatoes, raw	1 medium	0.2

FRUITS

Food	Portion	SF2
Prunes, canned	½ cup	1.5
Raisins, seedless	½ cup	1.5
Apple, with skin	1 medium	1.0
Applesauce, canned, unsweetened	½ cup	1.0
Apricots	3 apricots	1.0
Avocado	¼ of medium	1.0
Boysenberries, canned, water-pack	½ cup	1.0
Figs	1 medium	1.0
Pear	1 medium	1.0
Prunes, dried	3 prunes	1.0
Banana	1 medium	0.5
Blackberries	½ cup	0.5
Grapefruit	½ medium	0.5
Melon, cantaloupe, or honeydew	1 cup	0.5
Nectarine	1 small	0.5
Peach	1 medium	0.5
Plums	3 small	0.5

Food	Portion	SF2
Raspberries, canned, water-pack	½ cup	0.5
Strawberries	½ cup	0.5
Tangerine	1 small	0.5
Dates	2 dates	0.4
Blueberries	½ cup	0.3
Cherries, sweet	10 cherries	0.3
Orange	1 small	0.3
Pineapple	½ cup	0.3
Raspberries	½ cup	0.2
Grapes	12 grapes	0.1

NUTS

Food	Portion	SF2
Almonds	21 nuts	0.5
Brazil nuts	8 nuts	0.4
Hazelnuts (filberts)	21 nuts	0.4
Pecans	8 nuts	0.3
Walnuts	7 nuts	0 2
Peanut butter	2 tbsp	0 2
Peanut	32 nuts	0 0
Cashews	13 nuts	0.3
Macadamia nuts	11 nuts	0.8
Coconut meat	1 oz	1.2

DESSERTS AND SNACKS

Laboratory values for soluble fiber are not available for many of the foods in this category. In most cases, the SF2 values in this table are based on an assumption that 30 percent of the total dietary fiber is in the soluble form. The SF2 values of several foods in this table are based on typical recipes for those foods. These estimates are close enough to use for selecting foods to meet your daily goal for soluble fiber.

Food	Portion	SF2
Apple pie	⅙ of 9" pie	2.0
Oatmeal cookies	4, 2 5" diameter	1.5
Banana chocolate cream pie	⅙ of 9" pie	1.0
Cheesecake, graham cracker crust	⅛ cake	0.5
Chocolate chip cookies	4, 2.25" diameter	0.5
Gingerbread	⅑ of 8" cake	0.5

USING SF2

Food	Portion	SF2
Lemon meringue pie	⅙ of 9" pie	0.5
Brownie, chocolate, with icing	1, 1.5" x 1.75"	0.3
Devil's food cake, chocolate icing	⅟₁₆ of 9" cake	0.3
Popcorn, air-popped	1 cup	0.3
Popcorn, microwave-popped	1 cup	0.3
Popcorn, oil-popped	1 cup	0.3
Pound cake	⅟₁₇ of loaf	0.2
Sherbet, orange	1 cup	0.2
Angel food cake	⅟₁₂ of 10" cake	0.1
Chocolate, dark	1 oz.	0.1
Chocolate chips, chocolate flavored	¼ cup	0.1
Corn chips	1 oz.	0.1
Milk chocolate bar	1 oz.	0.1
Potato chips	1 oz.	0.1
Custard, from mix	½ cup	0.0
Chocolate pudding, 2% milk	½ cup	0.0
Ice cream, vanilla, 10% fat	1 cup	0.0
Ice cream, vanilla, 16% fat	1 cup	0.0
Ice milk, vanilla, hard	1 cup	0.0
Pretzels	1 oz.	0.0
Tapioca made with skim milk	½ cup	0.0
Gelatin	½ cup	0.0

BEVERAGES

Food	Portion	SF2
Apple juice	8 oz.	0.5
Tomato juice	8 oz.	0.5
Vegetable juice	8 oz.	0.5
Orange juice, fresh	8 oz.	0.3
Chocolate shake	10 oz.	0.2
Chocolate milk, 1% fat	8 oz.	0.1
Chocolate milk, whole milk	8 oz.	0.1
Hot chocolate, with whole milk	8 oz.	0.1
Coffee, black	8 oz.	0.0
Cola, regular	12 oz.	0.0
Ginger ale	12 oz.	0.0
Lemonade, from mix	8 oz.	0.0
Orange drink	8 oz.	0.0
Tea, without milk	8 oz.	0.0
Eggnog	8 oz.	0.0

FATS AND OILS
Fats and oils do not contain any soluble fiber.

GRAVIES, SAUCES, AND DRESSINGS
Gravies, sauces, and dressings contain only trace amounts of soluble fiber.

MISCELLANEOUS FOODS

Food	Portion	SF2
Psyllium flower supplement	1 tbsp.	3.0
Baking chocolate	1 oz.	0.2
Cocoa powder	2 tsp.	0.1
Spices and herbs	1 tsp.	0.1
Baking powder	1 tsp.	0.0
Half and half creamer	1 tbsp.	0.0
Nondairy creamer, powdered	1 tsp.	0.0
Pancake syrup	1 oz.	0.0
Tofu	5.5 oz.	0.0
Whipped topping, frozen	1 tbsp.	0.0

Remember, keep track of the foods you eat and the SF2 points that correspond to each of them—and choose enough foods with a high soluble-fiber content to reach your SF2 goal. Your daily objective is to eat enough grams of soluble fiber to equal or exceed your SF2 number (but don't go over 18 grams of soluble fiber a day).

Reaching your SF2 goal each day is really not difficult—in fact, it doesn't take any extra work if you make the right kinds of selections from the SF1 Lists in Chapter Eight. The fact is, high soluble fiber and low saturated fat go hand in hand—that is, the more careful you are about avoiding foods high in saturated fat, the more likely you are to select foods high in soluble fiber. To prove that point, let's review the menus that you saw in Chapter Eight. This time, we'll look at the SF2 values for the foods that were chosen.

Our first example in Chapter Eight was an inactive 190-pound male whose ideal weight is 160. Some very poor food selections caused his saturated-fat intake to far exceed his SF1 number. Using the SF2 chart, we determined that his personal SF2 number is 15. This is how his day's menu performed in the SF2 category:

	SF2 Value
Breakfast	
Eggs, soft-boiled (2)	0.0
Bacon, fried (3.5 oz.)	0.0
Whole wheat toast (2 slices)	0.6
with butter (1 tbsp.)	0.0
Coffee (2 cups)	0.0
with half-and-half creamer (1 tbsp.)	0.0
Lunch	
Bologna and cheese sandwich:	
Bologna (3 slices)	0.0
Whole-milk ricotta cheese (2 oz.)	0.0
Whole wheat bread (2 slices)	0.6
Lettuce	0.1
Mayonnaise (1 tsp.)	0.0
Potato chips (2 oz.)	0.2
Iced tea (8 oz.)	0.0
with sugar (2 tsp.)	0.0
Dinner	
Tossed salad:	
Lettuce (1 cup)	0.4
Tomato, onions	0.5
Pork spare ribs (7 oz.)	0.0
Baked potato (1)	2.0
with butter (1 tbsp.)	0.0
with sour cream (5 tbsp.)	0.0
Cooked vegetables (carrots, peas; 1 cup)	3.0
with butter (1 tbsp.)	0.0
Coffee (1 cup)	0.0
with half-and-half creamer (1 tbsp.)	0.0
Snacks, Desserts	
Lemon meringue pie (⅙ of 9" pie)	0.5
Cola drink	0.0
Total SF2 value for the day	7.9

This man's poor food choices are reflected in his SF2 total for the day, which falls far below his goal of 15.

The second case we examined was the same inactive male. But this time, he made some much healthier food choices. Using the SF2 chart, his personal SF2 goal is still 15. Let's look at his menu's soluble-fiber content:

	SF2 Value
Breakfast	
Oat bran cereal (1 cup)	2.0
Skim milk (8 oz.)	0.0
Grapefruit (½ medium)	0.5
Orange juice, fresh (8 oz.)	0.3
Oat bran and raisin muffin (1)	1.5
Coffee, decaf (1 cup)	0.0
Lunch	
Hamburger, lean (7 oz.) with bun, lettuce, tomato slice	0.6
with mayonnaise, imitation, soybean (1 tbsp.)	0.0
Split peas, cooked (½ cup)	1.5
Skim milk (8 oz.)	0.0
Pear (1 medium)	1.0
Iced tea	0.0
Dinner	
Halibut, broiled (7 oz.)	0.0
with lemon	0.0
Broccoli (½ cup)	1.0
Corn (½ cup)	1.5
Skim milk (8 oz.)	0.0
Snacks, Desserts	
Figs (5)	5.0
Cottage cheese, 1% fat (4 oz.)	0.0
Oat bran and raisin muffin (1)	1.5
Total SF2 value for the day	16.4

This time the man had no problem reaching his soluble fiber goal for the day at the same time he was cutting back on saturated fat.

Finally, here is the menu for the 128-pound moderately active woman; her ideal weight (120 pounds) gives her an SF2 number of 11. In Chapter Eight, we proposed the following food choices for her to keep her saturated-fat intake under her personal SF1 number. Now we'll examine them for soluble-fiber content:

	SF2 Value
Breakfast	
Oat bran cereal (½ cup)	1.0
with sliced banana (½ medium)	0.3
Skim milk (8 oz.)	0.0
Oat bran and raisin muffin (1)	1.5
Orange juice, fresh (8 oz.)	0.3
Coffee (1 cup)	0.0
with skim milk (1 oz.)	0.0
Lunch	
Soup, minestrone (1 cup)	1.0
Green salad (lettuce, chopped vegetables)	1.0
with Italian dressing (1 tbsp.)	0.0
Oat bran and raisin muffin (1)	1.5
Skim milk (8 oz.)	0.0
Dinner	
Chicken, light meat, no skin (3.5 oz.)	0.0
Steamed vegetables (1 cup: carrots, green beans)	1.5
Kidney beans (½ cup, cooked)	3.0
Coffee (1 cup)	0.0
with skim milk (1 oz.)	0.0
Snacks, Desserts	
Apple pie (1 slice)	2.0
Popcorn, air-popped (1 cup)	0.3
Total SF2 value for the day	13.4

As you can see, this woman exceeded her SF2 number (there is nothing wrong with that up to a maximum of 18 grams of soluble fiber per day). Her diet was varied, nutritious, and likely to be very satisfying.

As you make your own food choices, keep in mind what these sample menus have shown—namely, you can painlessly increase your soluble fiber intake and lower your saturated-fat consumption. And, by making food selections that head you in that direction, your cholesterol level will tend to drop, too.

GETTING A HEAD START
WITH OATS, BEANS, AND BLACK-EYED PEAS

The more varied your selection of high-fiber foods, the more you are likely to enjoy your cholesterol-lowering program and stick to it. But you can eliminate much of the work and worry about reaching your soluble-fiber goal by including a large portion each day of one of the foods "packed" with soluble fiber. Oat bran, beans, and black-eyed peas are worthy of special mention here because they are tasty, inexpensive, and can be used in a wide variety of ways. Here are a couple of hints to help you eat these foods regularly:

• Try to incorporate one-half to one cup of cooked dried beans or black-eyed peas into your meals each day. Serve them in combination with other foods as well as separately. By combining them with meats and poultry, you can "extend" those foods to help keep your saturated-fat intake low.

• Try incorporating oat bran into your diet in a variety of ways—in hot or cold cereal, in muffins or bread, in pancakes and waffles, even as a garnish on salads and other dishes. You'll find recipes for oat bran muffins on the boxes of most cereals that are high in oat bran.

FIBER SUPPLEMENTS

Soluble fiber is also abundantly available in another form—over-the-counter dietary fiber supplements. Though they were originally sold as a preventive measure against constipation, many are also very effective for lowering cholesterol levels. These supplements (with brand names like Metamucil, Fiberall, Correctol, Fiber Eze, Konsyl-D, and Hydrocil Instant) contain psyllium hydrophilic mucilloid, a natural soluble fiber that comes from the husks of blond psyllium seeds.

Several studies have documented the effectiveness of these fiber supplements as cholesterol-lowering agents. At the University of Kentucky, Dr. James Anderson placed thirteen men (cholesterol levels between 188 and 314) on 3.4 grams of psyllium three times a day. Another group of thirteen men was given a placebo, and both groups maintained their usual diets. After eight weeks, the total blood cholesterol level of the men taking psyllium had decreased an average of 15 percent, while their LDL had dipped 20 percent. No change was seen in HDL levels. Among the placebo group, no significant changes occurred in any cholesterol category. No one who took psyllium experienced any serious side effects, although some reported cramping or other mild gastrointestinal symptoms.

In 1988, Washington State University researchers published a study involving seven patients whose blood cholesterol levels ranged from 132 to 240. These individuals were given 21 grams per day of psyllium seed husks for three weeks. When blood cholesterol levels were checked ten days and three weeks after the supplementation began, cholesterol values had fallen significantly. Total cholesterol levels decreased by an average of 35 points at the ten-day cutoff, and settled in at a 30-point decline after three weeks. The higher the individual's starting cholesterol level, the greater the decrease that was experienced. In this study, however, HDL cholesterol levels fell along with the LDL.

It's important to remember that these studies are small ones, involving a limited number of patients. Even so, their findings are supported by about ten other small studies—some dating back to the 1960s—which have demonstrated drops in blood cholesterol of 55 to 20 percent when psyllium supplements (3.6 to 24.2 grams daily) were given. At the Wilhuri Research Institute in Helsinki, for instance, researchers gave psyllium husk to twelve elderly men and women. After ten weeks on the supplement, blood cholesterol levels had declined 20 percent. Most of these earlier studies, however, involved special types of patients, such as diabetics, obese individuals, and those in intensive care units.

How significant could these reductions be? Think back to the research cited in Chapter Two, noting that in people with high blood cholesterol levels, for each 1 percent decline in total cholesterol there was a 2 percent decrease in the risk of coronary heart disease. With that in mind, the 5 to 20 percent drops in total cholesterol levels in these studies could translate into significant reductions in the risk of heart attacks. The University of Kentucky researchers have called the fiber supplements "a safe, effective therapy" for treating high blood cholesterol levels.

But even though these supplements are loaded with fiber, their cost and their lack of other nutrients make them a clear second choice as a source of soluble fiber in a good diet. On the other hand, if you encounter some days when fiber-rich foods aren't easily available, the supplements

OTHER HEALTH BENEFITS OF FIBER

When you increase your intake of dietary fiber to lower your cholesterol, you receive some other health benefits as a bonus. To a great extent, these benefits occur because of the *insoluble* fiber that accompanies the soluble fiber in plant foods. Here are some of the things a high-fiber diet can accomplish:

• Fiber *may* decrease your risk of developing colon cancer. Fiber makes your stools move through the large intestine more rapidly; as a result, any cancer-causing agents in your stool have less time to create trouble in the lining of the colon. Some researchers also believe that the bulk which fiber adds to the stool dilutes any substances that may be cancer-causing. The evidence that a high-fiber diet will protect you against colon cancer is not yet conclusive, but a high-fiber diet is a prudent choice until the question is answered.

• Fiber can prevent constipation. As it moves through the large intestine, fiber attracts additional water into the stool, which softens it and speeds its elimination.

• Because of its laxative effect, fiber can reduce your chances of developing hemorrhoids (varicose veins of the rectum). Fiber makes the stools softer, which leads to less straining on the toilet and prevents excessive pressure on the rectal veins.

• If losing weight is one of your goals, a high-fiber diet may be a big help. When you eat a lot of fiber, the dietary bulk will give you a feeling of fullness more quickly than other foods do, thus discouraging overeating. Also, high-fiber foods—such as fruits and vegetables—tend to be low in calories.

can help you reach your SF2 quota. (By the way, as long as you are eating enough fiber to reach your SF2 number, constipation is one of the last things you will have to worry about!)

SIDE EFFECTS OF A HIGH-FIBER DIET

With all the good news about fiber, is there a downside to this food component? For some people, the answer is yes, but the side effects usually don't warrant a great deal of concern. Most commonly, eating foods such as beans tends to increase the amount of gas produced in the intestines.

Though initially disturbing (and embarrassing) to some people, this effect tends to taper off within a few weeks after adoption of a bean-rich diet. Also, in large quantities, dietary fiber causes some people to experience cramping or diarrhea. These complaints can usually be minimized if you increase your fiber intake gradually, adding just a few grams each day until you get up to your SF2 number. In almost all cases, the discomfort disappears within a few days, after your body has had a little time to get used to the higher fiber load. From the beginning, the intensity of these symptoms varies from person to person.

With fiber—as with so many other substances—you can get too much of a good thing. There is a possibility that at extremely high levels, certain minerals (magnesium, iron, selenium, copper, zinc, and calcium) might bind to the fiber, causing these essential minerals to be eliminated in the stool instead of being absorbed into the bloodstream. So while you should try to meet your SF2 number each day, it is not necessary or wise to overdo it.

Finally, there have been some reports of allergic reactions to psyllium, including sneezing, itchy eyes or nose, and a runny nose. These reported reactions have occurred primarily in workers who manufacture the psyllium products, but they apparently can also affect people who ingest the products.

HIGH-SOLUBLE-FIBER DISHES

As in Chapter Eight, we have a few recipes for you—this time for high-soluble-fiber dishes. Once again, they were created by the Good Housekeeping Institute. Try them all over the next few days and weeks, and make them a regular part of your meal planning.

- Black bean soup
- Fire alarm barley
- Mixed-fruit compote
- Oat bran and raisin muffins
- Oat bran and raisin cookies

Black Bean Soup

1 16-ounce package dry black beans
1 tablespoon salad oil
1 large onion, diced
1 large green pepper, diced
1 large garlic clove, minced
1 15-ounce can tomato sauce
2 teaspoons salt (optional)
1/2 teaspoon pepper

1. About 4 hours before serving, rinse beans with running cold water and discard any stones or shriveled beans. In 5-quart saucepot over high heat, heat beans and 8 cups water to boiling; boil 3 minutes. Remove saucepot from heat; cover and let beans stand 1 hour.

2. In 10-inch skillet over medium heat, in hot salad oil, cook onion, green pepper, and garlic until tender, stirring occasionally.

3. Stir onion mixture into undrained beans; add tomato sauce, salt, and pepper. Heat to boiling. Reduce heat to low; cover and simmer mixture about 2 hours, or until beans are tender, stirring occasionally.

Makes about 9 cups, or 9 servings. About 190 calories, 0 mg cholesterol per serving. SF1 value: 0.2; SF2 value: 3.5.

Fire Alarm Barley

1 cup barley
1/4 cup chili powder
1 tablespoon sugar
1 1/2 teaspoons salt (optional)
1 large garlic clove, minced
1/4 teaspoon hot pepper sauce
1 10-ounce package frozen peas

1. About 1 hour before serving, in 4-quart saucepot over high heat, heat barley, chili powder, sugar, salt, garlic, hot pepper sauce, and 3 cups water to boiling. Reduce heat to low; cover and simmer about 50 minutes, or until barley is tender and liquid is absorbed.

2. About 10 minutes before barley is done, stir in frozen peas.

Makes 8 servings. About 95 calories, 0 mg cholesterol per serving. SF1 value: 0.0; SF2 value: 1.5.

Mixed-Fruit Compote

1 12-ounce package dried Mission figs
1 12-ounce package pitted prunes
1 4-ounce package dried apple rings
3 cups orange juice

A day ahead, in heat-proof medium bowl, combine figs, prunes, and apple rings. In 2-quart saucepan over medium heat, heat orange juice to boiling. Pour orange juice over fruit in bowl. Cover, and refrigerate overnight. Stir before serving. Store fruit in refrigerator to use within 2 weeks.

Makes about 7 cups, or 14 servings. About 165 calories, 0 mg cholesterol per serving. SF1 value: 0.1; SF2 value: 2.5.

Oat Bran and Raisin Muffins

2 cups 100% oat bran, uncooked
2 teaspoons baking powder
1 teaspoon ground cinnamon
1/2 teaspoon ground nutmeg
1 cup skim milk
1/3 cup honey
1/4 cup salad oil
2 egg whites
1 cup dark seedless raisins

1. About 40 minutes before serving, or early in the day, preheat oven to 425°F. Place paper liners in twelve 2 1/2" by 1 1/4" muffin-pan cups.

2. In large bowl, mix first 4 ingredients. In small bowl, beat milk, honey, oil, and egg whites until blended; stir into oat bran mixture just until oat bran is moistened. Fold in raisins.

3. Spoon batter into cups to come almost to top of each cup. Bake 20 minutes, or until toothpick inserted in center of muffin comes out clean. Immediately remove muffins from pan; serve warm. Or cool them on a wire rack.

Makes 12 muffins. About 155 calories, negligible cholesterol per muffin. SF1 value: 1.0; SF2 value: 1.5.

Oat Bran and Raisin Cookies

Preheat oven to 350°F. Lightly grease cookie sheet. Prepare Oat Bran and Raisin Muffins recipe as above, but omit skim milk. Drop dough by level tablespoonfuls, about 2 inches apart, onto cookie sheet. Bake about 15 minutes, or until edges are lightly browned. With metal spatula, remove cookies to wire rack to cool. Repeat until all dough is used, lightly greasing cookie sheet each time.

Makes about 2 dozen cookies. About 75 calories, 0 mg cholesterol per cookie. SF1 value: 0.5; SF2 value: 0.5.

10

♥　♥　♥　♥

MORE STRATEGIES TO GET YOUR CHOLESTEROL DOWN

As you have already seen, our primary strategies for counting out cholesterol involve decreasing the amount of saturated fat you eat each day and increasing the amount of soluble fiber. These particular intake and absorption factors are likely to give you the greatest amount of cholesterol-lowering effect with the least effort and with minimal disruption of your lifestyle. But there are other strategies you can use to enhance your cardiovascular health, and you should take advantage of all of them. In this chapter, you will find three additional actions that can increase your chances for success. Each one is important. If you are not already doing them, now is the time to get started.

COUNT OUT DIETARY CHOLESTEROL

Although saturated fat is the major dietary contributor to high blood cholesterol, the cholesterol that is present in the foods you eat also plays a significant role. However essential cholesterol is for health, it is not an essential part of your diet. As you learned in Chapter Three, even if you ate no cholesterol, your liver would manufacture all the cholesterol your body needs. The dietary cholesterol you consume only sets you up for excess levels of cholesterol in your blood.

There is no cholesterol in plant foods like fruits, vegetables, and cereals, but dietary cholesterol is present in many of the other foods we eat, and it is difficult to avoid completely. It is found not only in animal tissues (meat, poultry, fish) but also in animal products such as milk, cheese, butter, and eggs. You do not need to avoid cholesterol entirely in order to lower your blood cholesterol level, but you do need to limit the amount you eat to less than 300 milligrams per day. (The average American consumes about 350 to 450 milligrams of cholesterol per day.)

Cholesterol and saturated fat tend to go hand in hand—foods that are low in saturated fat also tend to be low in cholesterol, and foods that are high in one are likely to be high in the other. There are some exceptions to this general rule, and it's important to be aware of them so they don't spoil the effect of the other cholesterol-reducing efforts you are making. For example, although liver is low in saturated fat (less than 2 grams in a 3.5 ounce portion), it is extremely high in cholesterol—almost 400 milligrams of cholesterol are present in the same-size portion. Shrimp also stands out: 3.5 ounces of this shellfish contain less than 1 gram of saturated fat and almost 200 milligrams of cholesterol. Of course, the best-known high-cholesterol culprit is the egg. An average egg has less than 2 grams of saturated fat—but more than 270 milligrams of cholesterol. Eat just one egg, and you have almost filled your entire cholesterol quota for the day.

Actually, it's the egg yolk, not the white, that contains the cholesterol. So although you should limit the number of *whole* eggs you eat, there is no need to slow down your consumption of *whites* (this part of the egg contains no cholesterol at all). Many people discard the yolks before they cook eggs, and find—often to their surprise—that the egg whites retain much of the "eggy" flavor. Try it yourself—use just the whites to make an omelette or scrambled eggs.

As you try to curtail your egg intake, keep in mind that egg yolks are used in the manufacture of many processed and cooked food products. For most people, the majority of their egg consumption comes from the "invisible" eggs that are parts of foods such as pancakes or French toast. Eggs are also often included in breads, cakes, cookies, ice cream, mayonnaise, meat loaf, pastas, puddings, quiche, and salad dressings, so these foods should be eaten in thoughtful quantities. Do your shopping carefully, too. Read the label of every product you buy at the market and you'll discover dozens of eggs that you never realized you were eating. Incidentally, commercial egg substitutes—which do not contain yolks— are acceptable alternatives to eating natural eggs. They are made almost exclusively from egg whites, along with a small amount of fat.

In addition to eggs, you also should carefully control the amount of organ meat you consume. If you are one of those people who still enjoys an occasional course of liver and onions, keep it only occasional, because a single 3.5-ounce serving will exceed your total allowance of cholesterol for the day. Other organ meats—including brain, heart, tongue, kidneys, sweetbreads (thymus), and chitterlings—fare no better, with most having between 180 and 470 milligrams of cholesterol in a 3.5-ounce serving. And if you think that chicken liver might be an acceptable alternative to beef liver, think again. Chicken liver has 631 milligrams of cholesterol per 3.5-ounce serving!

Keeping your cholesterol intake under 300 milligrams per day is not as difficult as it sounds. In fact, if you adhere conscientiously to your daily SF1 goal, your intake of dietary cholesterol will probably fall automatically under 300.

The lists that follow will show you the cholesterol content of the foods listed in Chapters Eight and Nine. If you don't exceed your SF1 quota for saturated fat each day, and if you cut way back on the foods that are very high in dietary cholesterol, there is no need to count the precise amount of cholesterol you eat each day. Even so, some people find it valuable to do so for just a few days as they get started on this program, just to get a better appreciation for how much cholesterol they've been eating in the past.

Chart 20

CHOLESTEROL VALUES OF FOODS

The following tables list the amount of cholesterol per portion (in milligrams) for commonly used foods. If your portion is larger or smaller, you will have to multiply or divide the value accordingly. These numbers have been rounded off to the nearest 10 milligrams, except when the amount of cholesterol in a portion is 5 milligrams or less, in which case the actual value is reported. While these values are approximations, they are accurate enough to help you determine your cholesterol intake.

The more foods you choose from the top of each table, and the less you eat of foods at the bottom, the more your blood cholesterol level is likely to drop.

MEATS

Food	Portion	Chol
Sausage, pork	2 links	20
Ham slices, lean	2 slices	30
Salami, beef	2 slices	30
Smoked ham	3.5 oz	60
Bologna, beef	3-4 slices	60
Frankfurter, beef	2 franks	60
Sausage, beef	2 links	70
Round, beef, lean	3.5 oz	80
Tenderloin, lean	3.5 oz	80
T-bone, lean	3.5 oz	80
Leg of lamb, lean	3.5 oz	90
Sirloin, lean	3.5 oz	90
Ground beef, lean	3.5 oz	90
Ribs, lean	3.5 oz	90
Bacon, fried	3.5 oz	90
Corned beef	3.5 oz	100
Lamb chop, lean	3.5 oz	110
Spare ribs, pork	3.5 oz	120
Veal cutlet, medium fat	3.5 oz	130
Kidneys, simmered	3.5 oz	390
Liver, braised	3.5 oz	390

POULTRY

Food	Portion	Chol
Turkey roll	3 slices	40
Bologna, turkey	3 slices	60
Chicken, light meat, no skin	3.5 oz	80
Frankfurter, turkey	2 franks	80
Chicken, dark meat, no skin	3.5 oz	90
Turkey, light meat, no skin	3.5 oz	90
Duck, no skin	3.5 oz	90
Frankfurter, chicken	2 franks	90
Turkey, dark meat, no skin	3.5 oz	110

SEAFOOD

Food	Portion	Chol
Anchovies, canned, in oil	5 anchovies	17
Tuna, albacore, canned, water-pack	3.5 oz	30
Perch	3.5 oz	40
Halibut	3.5 oz	40
Rockfish	3.5 oz	40
Snapper	3.5 oz	50
Grouper	3.5 oz	50
Sea bass	3.5 oz	50
Swordfish	3.5 oz	50
Tuna, bluefin	3.5 oz	50
Cod	3.5 oz	60
Mussels	3.5 oz	60
Pompano	3.5 oz	60
Lobster	3.5 oz	70
Clams	3.5 oz	70
Haddock	3.5 oz	70
Trout	3.5 oz	70
Herring	3.5 oz	80
Mackerel	3.5 oz	80
Salmon	3.5 oz	90
Crab	3.5 oz	100
Pollock	3.5 oz	100
Oysters	3.5 oz	110
Shrimp	3.5 oz	160
Eel	3.5 oz	200

DAIRY PRODUCTS

Food	Portion	Chol
Egg, white	1	0
Yogurt, plain, nonfat	8 oz.	4
Skim milk	8 oz.	4
Parmesan cheese, grated	1 tbsp.	4
Cottage cheese, 1% fat	4 oz.	5
Buttermilk	8 oz.	10
Low-fat milk, 1% fat	8 oz.	10
Yogurt, flavored, low-fat	8 oz.	10
American processed cheese slices	1 oz. (1.5 slices)	20
American processed cheese spread	1 oz.	20
Cottage cheese, creamed	4 oz.	20
Low-fat milk, 2% fat	8 oz.	20
Mozzarella, part-skim	1 oz.	20
Cheese, whole-milk	1 oz.	30
Whole milk, 3.3% fat	8 oz.	30
Yogurt, plain, whole milk	8 oz.	30
Ricotta, part-skim	4 oz.	30
Cream cheese	1 oz.	30
Butter	1 tbsp.	30
Ricotta, whole-milk	4 oz.	60
Egg, whole	1	270
Quiche	⅛ of 8" diameter	290

GRAINS, PASTA, RICE, AND PIZZA

Food	Portion	Chol
Bulgur wheat, cooked	1 cup	0
Barley, pearled	2 tbsp.	0
Cornmeal, degermed	1 cup	0
Flour, all-purpose or whole wheat	1 cup	0
Flour, wheat, cake	1 cup	0
Macaroni, cooked	1 cup	0
Spaghetti, cooked	1 cup	0
Rice, brown, cooked	1 cup	0
Rice, white, instant, cooked	1 cup	0
Noodles, chow mein	1 cup	0
Pizza, cheese	⅛ of 15" pie	20
Egg noodles, cooked	1 cup	50

SOUPS

Food	Portion	Chol
Vegetables, canned	1 cup	0
Black bean, canned, made with water	1 cup	0
Gazpacho	1 cup	0
Onion, made with water	1 cup	0
Beef bouillon, canned	1 cup	0
Tomato, made with water	1 cup	0
Chicken broth, canned, made with water	1 cup	1
Cream of mushroom, canned, made with water	1 cup	2
Minestrone	1 cup	5
Split pea with ham	1 cup	10
Chicken noodle, canned, made with water	1 cup	10
Cream of chicken, canned, made with water	1 cup	10
Beef, chunky, canned	1 cup	10
Clam chowder, Manhattan style	1 cup	10
Clam chowder, New England style, with skim milk	1 cup	20
Tomato, made with skim milk	1 cup	20
Cream of mushroom, made with skim milk	1 cup	20
Chicken, chunky, canned	1 cup	30
Cream of chicken, canned, made with skim milk	1 cup	30

BREADS AND CRACKERS

Food	Portion	Chol
Oat bran and raisin muffins, our recipe	1 muffin	0
Oat bran bread	1 slice	0
Tortilla, corn	1 tortilla	0
Pita bread, white	½ large shell	0
Bagel, plain	1, 3.5" diameter	0
English muffin	1 muffin	0
Hamburger bun	1 bun	0
White bread, enriched	1 slice	0
Whole wheat bread	1 slice	0
Frankfurter bun	1 bun	0
Graham crackers	2 squares	0
Whole wheat crackers	5 crackers	0
Melba toast, plan	1 piece	0
Saltines	1 cracker	0
Croissant	1, 4.5" x 4"	10

Food	Portion	Chol
Corn muffin	1, 2.5" diameter	20
Pancakes, made with skim milk	1, 4" diameter	20
Doughnut, plain	1, 3.25" diameter	20
Bran muffin	1, 2.5" diameter	20
Waffle, plain, dry mix, complete	1 waffle	38

CEREALS

Pure grain products, including cereals, do not contain any cholesterol. If cereal is eaten with milk, the cholesterol content of the milk must be considered.

BEANS

Beans do not contain any cholesterol.

VEGETABLES

Vegetables do not contain any cholesterol.

FRUITS

Fruits do not contain any cholesterol.

NUTS

Nuts do not contain any cholesterol.

DESSERTS AND SNACKS

Food	Portion	Chol
Apple pie	⅙ of 9" pie	0
Chocolate chips, chocolate flavored	¼ cup	0
Chocolate, dark	1 oz.	0
Angel food cake	1/12 of 10" cake	0
Potato chips	1 oz.	0
Gelatin	½ cup	0
Pretzels	1 oz.	0
Popcorn, oil-popped	1 cup	0
Popcorn, microwave-popped	1 cup	0
Popcorn, air-popped	1 cup	0
Corn chips	1 oz.	0
Gingerbread	⅑ of 8" cake	1
Oatmeal cookies	4, 2.5" diameter	2

Food	Portion	Chol
Chocolate pudding, 2% milk	½ cup	9
Banana chocolate cream pie	⅙ of 9" pie	10
Brownie, chocolate, with icing	1, 1.5" x 1.75"	10
Milk chocolate	1 oz.	10
Sherbet, orange	1 cup	10
Chocolate chip cookies	4, 2.25" diameter	20
Tapioca, made with skim milk	½ cup	20
Ice milk, vanilla, hard	1 cup	20
Cheesecake, graham cracker crust	⅛ cake	30
Devil's food cake, chocolate icing	¹⁄₁₆ of 9" cake	40
Pound cake	¹⁄₁₇ of loaf	60
Ice cream, vanilla, 10% fat	1 cup	60
Custard, from mix	½ cup	80
Ice cream, vanilla, 16% fat	1 cup	90
Lemon meringue pie	⅙ of 9" pie	140

BEVERAGES

Food	Portion	Chol
Apple juice	8 oz.	0
Tomato juice	8 oz.	0
Vegetable juice	8 oz.	0
Orange juice, fresh	8 oz.	0
Coffee, black	8 oz.	0
Cola, regular	12 oz.	0
Ginger ale	12 oz.	0
Lemonade, from mix	8 oz.	0
Orange drink	8 oz.	0
Tea, without milk	8 oz.	0
Chocolate milk, 1% fat	8 oz.	10
Chocolate milk, whole milk	8 oz.	30
Hot chocolate, with whole milk	8 oz.	30
Chocolate shake	10 oz.	40
Eggnog	8 oz.	150

FATS AND OILS

Food	Portion	Chol
Cooking spray, cholesterol-free	2-sec. spray	0
Safflower oil	1 tbsp.	0
Canola oil	1 tbsp.	0

COUNT OUT CHOLESTEROL

Food	Portion	Chol
Corn oil	1 tbsp.	0
Sunflower oil	1 tbsp.	0
Margarine, soft, tub	1 tbsp.	0
Imitation margarine, soft, tub	1 tbsp.	0
Olive oil	1 tbsp.	0
Sesame oil	1 tbsp.	0
Soybean oil	1 tbsp.	0
Peanut oil	1 tbsp.	0
Shortening	1 tbsp.	0
Cottonseed oil	1 tbsp.	0
Palm oil	1 tbsp.	0
Palm kernel oil	1 tbsp.	0
Coconut oil	1 tbsp.	0
Imitation mayonnaise, soybean	1 tbsp.	4
Mayonnaise	1 tbsp.	10
Lard	1 tbsp.	10
Butter	1 tbsp.	30

GRAVIES, SAUCES, AND DRESSINGS

Food	Portion	Chol
Sweet and sour sauce	½ cup	0
Barbecue sauce	½ cup	0
Au jus gravy, canned	½ cup	1
Turkey gravy, canned	½ cup	3
Chicken gravy, canned	½ cup	3
Beef gravy, canned	½ cup	4
Sour cream	1 tbsp.	5
White sauce	½ cup	20
Cheese sauce	½ cup	30
Hollandaise sauce	½ cup	90
Béarnaise sauce	½ cup	100
Italian dressing	1 tbsp.	0
Salad dressing, low-calorie	1 tbsp.	1
French dressing	1 tbsp.	1
Russian dressing	1 tbsp.	3
Blue cheese dressing	1 tbsp.	3
Thousand Island dressing	1 tbsp.	4

MISCELLANEOUS FOODS

Food	Portion	Chol
Tofu	5.5 oz.	0
Psyllium flower supplement	1 tbsp.	0
Cocoa powder	2 tsp.	0
Baking chocolate	1 oz.	0
Spices and herbs	1 tsp.	0
Baking powder	1 tsp.	0
Pancake syrup	1 oz.	0
Nondairy creamer, powdered	1 tsp.	0
Whipped topping, frozen	1 tbsp.	1
Half & half creamer	1 tbsp.	10

STRATEGIES FOR COUNTING UP ON HDL

In Part One of this book, you learned of the "protective" properties of HDL cholesterol (the so-called "good" cholesterol). The higher you can get your HDL level, the lower your risk of coronary heart disease. You do not have to sit back and hope for that to happen—there are some specific actions you can take to help increase your HDL level. Though these activities are not likely to produce as large a shift in HDL levels as dietary changes can produce in LDL levels, any increase in the HDL level—no matter how small—should be welcomed.

Exercising for a Higher HDL

While the increases in HDL caused by exercise tend to be modest, there is good reason to believe that they are very significant when it comes to preventing coronary heart disease. One thing is certain—regular exercise makes HDL levels go up.

Researchers with the Lipid Research Clinics reported on the experience of 4,386 men and women aged twenty years and older. When adjusted for any other factor that might influence HDL levels (including cigarette smoking and alcohol use), their findings showed that participants who reported some strenuous physical activity generally had higher HDL levels than their counterparts who reported no such exercise.

Active men, for instance, had an average HDL of 47.1, compared to 45.2 for inactive men. The active women had HDLs averaging 59.6, almost two points higher than sedentary females (57.7).

At Stanford University, researchers compared the cholesterol levels of men and women runners (who averaged fifteen miles a week or more) to those of people who got no exercise. They found that in the runners, a much larger proportion of the blood cholesterol was HDL. The ratio of total cholesterol to HDL was 3:1 in the runners (a very desirable ratio—see Chapter Five), compared to 4.9:1 in the sedentary subjects. The high-intensity exercise produced significant improvements in these individuals.

However, you don't have to be a runner to reap benefits from physical activity. Many researchers have found that less strenuous exercise can be just as helpful. A study in Oregon, published in 1983, examined eight patients who had high total blood cholesterol levels but very low HDL levels. They were placed on an eight-week walking program, with most subjects walking ten to thirty miles per week. As a result, the HDL levels in this group increased from an average of 31 to 35—a modest but still statistically significant change for the better.

In 1988, Brown University researchers reported a study in which eight previously sedentary men with desirable blood cholesterol levels (average 172) were placed on an exercise program involving an hour a day of stationary cycling. After fourteen weeks, HDL levels increased from an average of 37 to 42.

In one study, when overweight people participated in an exercise program, not only did they tend to lose weight, but their HDL levels increased in the process, particularly when they combined exercise with good eating habits. Dr. Peter Wood of Stanford University and his colleagues placed moderately overweight volunteers on a low-fat, low-cholesterol diet. Some of them adopted a walking or jogging program as well. After a year, HDL levels rose in men and women who adhered to both the exercise and the dietary plans. The combination of both diet and exercise had a more positive effect on HDL, LDL, and triglyceride levels than diet alone.

Thus, HDL cholesterol isn't the only component of blood cholesterol improved by an active lifestyle. By exercising regularly, you may also decrease your LDL (the so-called "bad" cholesterol). There is some debate whether this decline is a direct result of the exercise itself or rather a consequence of the weight loss that often accompanies an exercise program (overweight people tend to lower their LDL cholesterol levels as they shed excess pounds). Whatever the reason, the decrease in LDL is a highly desirable outcome.

What type of exercise is best? Several studies show that endurance athletes have HDL measurements 10 to 24 points higher than sedentary individuals. But, as the Oregon and Brown University studies involving walkers and cyclists demonstrate, you do not have to become an exercise fanatic to get cholesterol benefits; even a moderate amount of "aerobic" activity will be helpful. By definition, aerobic activities are those that cause the heart to beat faster and the lungs to breathe in more air for an extended time period. And there are many activities that meet this criteria. Here are some of the best aerobic exercises:

Brisk walking
Swimming
Jogging
Indoor (stationary) cycling or outdoor bicycling
Racquetball
Cross-country skiing
Indoor (or outdoor) rowing
Aerobic dance

With guidance from your physician, you should select an aerobic exercise that you are willing to commit yourself to for the next thirty days. To gain the full cardiovascular benefits, you will need to exercise about a half-hour at least three times per week (preferably more). That's not asking a lot to reduce your risk of a heart attack.

Be sure to choose an exercise that you will enjoy, or—better yet—rotate among several different aerobic activities to keep your exercise from getting boring. If you are not sure what exercise to do—choose walking. It's an activity that will raise your heart rate, it's free and requires no special equipment, and it's fun to do. If you haven't exercised regularly, start out slowly with a twenty-to-thirty-minute walk (one to two miles) every other day. Then gradually increase your distance and your pace until you are covering three miles, four to five times a week, in forty-five minutes or less. Give yourself as much time as it takes to get up to this distance and pace—even if it takes months. The earlier you start, the sooner you'll be able to start counting *up* on HDL. But particularly if you have been sedentary in recent months, talk with your doctor before beginning any exercise program.

Cigarettes: Calling It Quits

You almost certainly know that cigarettes are bad for your health. But as familiar as you probably are with the association between smoking and cancer—particularly lung cancer—you may be less acquainted with the link between cigarettes and blood cholesterol. The message is simple. Smoking dramatically increases the risk of coronary heart disease, at least in part by causing HDL levels to go down.

The Lipid Research Clinics program studied more than 5,200 men and women (ages 20 to 69) and found that smokers had significantly lower HDL cholesterol levels than did nonsmokers. The effect was directly related to the level of cigarette smoking—in this study, heavy smokers had lower HDL levels than light smokers. Once researchers had adjusted for four other factors that could influence blood cholesterol (alcohol intake, exercise, obesity, age), they found that heavy male smokers had an average HDL cholesterol of 40.9, compared to 46.2 in male nonsmokers. Many other studies back up these findings.

You won't be surprised, then, by this recommendation: If you smoke, you need to quit. Even if you've smoked for twenty years, thirty years, or more, it is never too late to stop. Your risk of heart disease will begin to drop almost immediately after you've kicked the habit, and once you have been a nonsmoker for more than a year, your HDL value will be approximately that of someone who has never smoked.

If you can't stop smoking on your own, ask your doctor to help you, or join one of the many excellent (and low-cost) classes conducted by the American Heart Association, the American Cancer Society, and the American Lung Association. Call the local branch of any of these organizations, and they will tell you when the next class starts.

Alcohol

There is some evidence that alcohol can raise the HDL cholesterol level and perhaps protect against heart attacks. The Honolulu Heart Study examined about 7,700 Japanese men living in Hawaii and in 1977 reported that those men who consumed a drink or two a day had a lower rate of heart attacks than the teetotalers.

A 1992 study hypothesized that although the population in France consumes large amounts of saturated fat, it has a low death rate from coronary heart disease, perhaps because of their high wine consumption; in this study, however, the effect of moderate alcohol intake on HDL cholesterol was considered only a partial explanation for alcohol's capacity to protect against heart disease.

Other studies have confirmed the fact that alcohol does raise HDL levels, but are less clear about the ultimate effect on the rate of heart attacks. One reason for the confusion is that there are several different subtypes of HDL, and no one is certain yet whether alcohol increases the level of the subtype (HDL-2) that is believed to be responsible for protecting against heart disease. Further research will have to be done before that question is answered.

In the meantime, few physicians are willing to recommend that you deliberately drink alcohol—a powerful drug—for the purpose of raising your HDL levels. The potential risks of alcohol use can hardly justify prescribing it for this purpose. If you do not already drink alcohol, you should not start drinking now with the idea of helping your heart. If you do drink, do not drink to excess for the purpose of increasing your HDL level. Heavy alcohol consumption has not been shown to be more effective for this purpose than light to moderate drinking (one or two drinks per day). It is hoped that future studies will provide more data about the relationship between alcohol, HDL levels, and the rate of heart attacks.

11

♥ ♥ ♥ ♥

MONITORING YOUR PROGRESS

You now have the information you need to begin your cholesterol-lowering program. Your personal SF1 and SF2 numbers
give you clear-cut targets to aim for each day. The food lists in
Chapters Eight and Nine will help you reach your goals for saturated fat
and soluble fiber, and the food lists in Chapter Ten will help you control
your intake of dietary cholesterol each day. It is time to put these tools to
work for you.

It is not easy to change a lifetime pattern of eating. To be successful,
you will need to pay special attention for a while to your food selections.
In time, healthier food choices will come automatically to you. To help
yourself get started, use the thirty-day diary you will find in this chapter.
The diary is an excellent tool for focusing your attention on what you are
eating. Using the diary will help you identify new foods and behaviors
that work especially well for you. This will enable you to develop a
cholesterol-lowering program that is specifically tailored to your personal tastes and desires. Such a program is likely not only to be more effective but also to afford more enjoyment to your eating.

♥♥♥♥♥♥♥♥♥♥♥♥♥♥♥
DAY 1
♥♥♥♥♥♥♥♥♥♥♥♥♥♥♥

Food	SF1 Value	SF2 Value	Cholesterol
Daily Total			

The diary can also be very helpful if your blood cholesterol level fails to respond well to the dietary changes you make initially. Your physician or dietician can use the diary to review the foods you have been eating, and to make recommendations for changes that may produce better results.

To gain maximum benefit from the diary, you should not let a day pass without entering your food choices, and determining whether you have met your goals for saturated fat, soluble fiber, and dietary cholesterol. If practical, carry this book with you throughout the day, and make your diary entries as you take your meals. That will ensure that your entries are complete and accurate. You'll also have the food lists handy in case questions arise about which foods to eat. If it is not practical to carry the book with you, keep notes throughout the day of the foods you eat, and translate them into diary entries before you go to bed. Take time then to review your day's food choices and to determine what foods you will eat the next day.

If you are one of those people who have difficulty writing in a book, or if this is a library book, make photocopies of the diary pages. Do this also if you wish to continue keeping a diary after the first thirty days are completed.

On the left-hand pages of this chapter, you will also find many helpful hints about low-cholesterol food choices and meal preparation. Read through them all now. Then review them again—one item at a time—as you make your entries each day in the diary. As much as you can, try to put these ideas into practice. The more you do, the more enjoyable and effective this program can be for you.

♥♥♥♥♥♥♥♥♥♥♥♥♥♥♥
DAY 2
♥♥♥♥♥♥♥♥♥♥♥♥♥♥♥

Food	SF1 Value	SF2 Value	Cholesterol
Daily Total			

FISH: MORE THAN JUST A MEAT SUBSTITUTE

Fish has suddenly become fashionable in the fight against heart disease, thanks to the Eskimos of Greenland, who eat lots of whale blubber and seal meat—both very high in fat—yet have a low incidence of heart attacks. Their healthy hearts are due, at least in part, to the fact that these fish fats are rich in a particular kind of oil called "omega-3 fatty acids." These fish oils apparently interfere slightly with the blood-clotting mechanism—just enough to reduce the likelihood of clots forming in the coronary arteries and causing heart attacks.

But that's not the only benefit these fish oils provide. There is some evidence to suggest that omega-3 fatty acids may have a direct effect which lowers LDL cholesterol and triglyceride levels in the blood. In one study at the Oregon Health Sciences University, volunteers fed a diet rich in fish (salmon) oils experienced a decline in total blood cholesterol levels from 188 to 162 and a drop in triglyceride levels from 77 to 48 over a four-week period. HDL concentrations remained unchanged.

The best source of omega-3 fish oils is cold-water marine fish. Here is a list of some of the best sources of these oils. Eating these fish about three times a week should give you a reasonable dose of omega-3 fatty acids.

Sources of Omega-3 Fish Oil

Bluefish	Herring	Smelt
Cod	Mackerel	Trout
Flounder	Salmon	Tuna
Haddock	Sardines	
Halibut	Shrimp	

Substituting 3 1/2 ounces of halibut for lean ground beef reduces the amount of saturated fat you eat by 6.8 grams and the cholesterol by 46 milligrams.

♥♥♥♥♥♥♥♥♥♥♥♥♥♥♥
DAY 3
♥♥♥♥♥♥♥♥♥♥♥♥♥♥♥

Food	SF1 Value	SF2 Value	Cholesterol
Daily Total			

FISH OIL CAPSULES:
DON'T MESS WITH MOTHER NATURE

Once the Eskimo-and-fish-oil story got out, it was just a matter of time until fish oil capsules began to appear on the shelves of America's pharmacies and health food stores. You can't blame people for trying them. After all, if a little fish oil is good for you, a little more ought to be better.

Unfortunately, things don't always work out that way. In fact, some studies have shown that these supplements may actually increase LDL levels rather than decrease them. In patients studied by University of Kansas researchers, thirteen of eighteen experienced a rise of more than 5 percent in LDL levels after taking fish oil capsules. This occurrence could not be explained, but another researcher may have found the reason why some fish oil capsules raised blood cholesterol levels—the capsules were loaded with cholesterol and saturated fat.

Until more research is done into the claims and potential adverse side effects of fish oil capsules, their value should be considered unproven and their use should be thought of as experimental. For now, if you want to increase your intake of omega-3 fatty acids, the best way to do it is by eating cold-water marine fish.

Substituting 3 1/2 ounces of salmon for 3 1/2 ounces of spareribs reduces the amount of saturated fat you eat by 9.9 grams and the cholesterol by 34 milligrams, and provides you with 1.3 grams of omega-3 fatty acids.

♥♥♥♥♥♥♥♥♥♥♥♥♥♥♥
DAY 4
♥♥♥♥♥♥♥♥♥♥♥♥♥♥♥

Food	SF1 Value	SF2 Value	Cholesterol
Daily Total			

CAN YOU DRINK CREAM AND BUTTERMILK?

Cream and half-and-half are both high in saturated fat. Surprisingly, so too are some nondairy creamers, although they are often advertised as a healthy alternative to cream for your coffee. Some of these products contain large amounts of coconut oil, which is a highly saturated fat.

To confuse matters, the labels of these nondairy creamers may accurately specify that they're free of cholesterol. That doesn't change the fact that your body will use the saturated fat in the creamer to make excess cholesterol. When selecting a nondairy creamer, look for one made from polyunsaturated fat (soybean, corn oil, safflower, sunflower). Other alternatives: Use skim milk in your coffee or drink it black.

Despite its name, there should be no butter in buttermilk. However, depending on its source, there can be a significant amount of fat. Buttermilk made from skim milk contains almost no fat (this is the kind you should look for). But buttermilk can also be made from low-fat or whole milk—in which case the saturated-fat content will be significant—and some dairies may add cream or butter chips to elevate the fat content. Always read the label before buying buttermilk to determine the actual fat content of the product you are considering.

Substituting one cup of skim milk for one cup of whole milk reduces the amount of saturated fat you eat by 4.7 grams and the cholesterol by 26 milligrams.

♥♥♥♥♥♥♥♥♥♥♥♥♥♥♥♥
DAY 5
♥♥♥♥♥♥♥♥♥♥♥♥♥♥♥♥

Food	SF1 Value	SF2 Value	Cholesterol
Daily Total			

CHOOSING AND USING YOGURT

Yogurt is high in nutritional value, and it can be low in fat and calories—but only if you select the right kind. The amount of saturated fat in yogurt varies widely according to which variety you buy. A cup of plain nonfat yogurt has 0.3 gram of saturated fat, a cup of low-fat has 2.3 grams, while whole-milk yogurt has 4.8 grams per cup. So the nonfat yogurt is a better choice than the low-fat, and both of these options are better than yogurt made from whole milk. Most supermarkets offer all varieties, so read the labels carefully before you put yogurt in your shopping cart.

Yogurt can help you keep your meals feeling "rich" without all the fat that usually goes along with that feeling. Here are some ways to use nonfat or low-fat yogurt in your cholesterol-lowering program:

- In place of high-fat salad dressings
- As a substitute for butter on baked potatoes
- As a dip for raw vegetables instead of sour cream (mix ing it with herbs and spices will give you the same good taste and feel that sour cream provides)
- As a tasty spread on bread and toast, especially when combined with crushed fresh fruit.

Substituting 8 ounces of low-fat yogurt for one cup of rich vanilla ice cream reduces the amount of saturated fat you eat by 14.5 grams and the cholesterol by 84 milligrams.

♥♥♥♥♥♥♥♥♥♥♥♥♥♥♥
DAY 6
♥♥♥♥♥♥♥♥♥♥♥♥♥♥♥

Food	SF1 Value	SF2 Value	Cholesterol
Daily Total			

BUTTER VS. MARGARINE

The taste of butter is very appealing, but you pay a very high price for it in terms of saturated fat and cholesterol. (Margarine can have about 70 percent less saturated fat, and has no cholesterol.) A tablespoon of butter has 31 milligrams of cholesterol and 7.6 grams of saturated fat. By comparison, a tablespoon of soft tub margarine has no cholesterol and only 1.8 grams of saturated fat. Making the switch has a real payoff.

You don't have to give up butter forever, but you should learn to use it less often and more sparingly. Save butter for when it counts—for example, to spread on a piece of good French bread in a fine restaurant. But don't drown waffles and potatoes in butter—the difference in taste between butter and margarine is not going to show through anyway.

There are many kinds of margarine to choose from, but some are not much better than butter itself, because the vegetable fats in them are saturated. So read the label carefully, and here is what to look for. Whether you're buying stick or tub margarine, select one with a liquid polyunsaturated oil (safflower, sunflower, corn, soybean) as the first ingredient on the label. This should guarantee that the product has more polyunsaturated than saturated oil. Also, choose a margarine that contains partially hydrogenated oils, not hydrogenated, and stay away from any margarines that contain coconut oil, palm oil, or lard.

Try to find an indication on the label that the margarine has at least twice as much polyunsaturated (P) as saturated (S) fat. On many labels, you'll find this information in the so-called P/S ratio; if it's two to one or greater, you've made a good choice.

Substituting one tablespoon of safflower tub margarine for one tablespoon of corn stick margarine reduces the amount of saturated fat you eat by .6 gram. Neither form of margarine has any cholesterol.

♥♥♥♥♥♥♥♥♥♥♥♥♥♥♥
DAY 7
♥♥♥♥♥♥♥♥♥♥♥♥♥♥♥

Food	SF1 Value	SF2 Value	Cholesterol
Daily Total			

MAKING THE MOST OF FRUITS AND VEGETABLES

Here's a simple rule that will help you select foods for your cholesterol-lowering program: Fruits or vegetables should be part of almost every meal. They are low in fat and high in fiber, they are good sources of vitamins and minerals, and they are low in calories. (As an additional bonus, there are studies that indicate that some yellow and green vegetables may help to protect against certain types of cancers.)

There are a few plant foods with which you must exert caution. Coconuts and avocados are both high in saturated fat. You don't have to give up these tasty choices completely, but you should learn to eat them only occasionally.

Although fresh fruits and vegetables are the ideal choice, there is nothing wrong with the frozen variety as far as its cholesterol-lowering value goes. If you do eat canned fruit, choose a brand that's packed in its own juice, not in a sugary syrup.

When preparing vegetables, you must be careful not to destroy their cholesterol-reducing value by drowning them in butter or margarine or blanketing them with sauces that are high in saturated fat and cholesterol. Besides, these things cover up the interesting natural taste of such foods. If you do want to give vegetables a little added flavor, try herbs, spices, lemon juice, or nonfat yogurt as toppings instead.

Substituting one medium apple for a slice of lemon meringue pie (1/6 of a 9-inch pie) reduces the amount of saturated fat you eat by 4.4 grams and the cholesterol by 143 milligrams.

♥♥♥♥♥♥♥♥♥♥♥♥♥♥♥♥
DAY 8
♥♥♥♥♥♥♥♥♥♥♥♥♥♥♥♥

Food	SF1 Value	SF2 Value	Cholesterol
Daily Total			

BREADS, CEREALS, AND COMPLEX CARBOHYDRATES

There was a time when steak and potatoes were considered the all-American dinner. How times change! Now that we understand the value of complex carbohydrates, spaghetti, macaroni, vegetable soups, and bread have taken important positions on the dinner table again. And rightfully so. These foods are generally high in fiber and low in saturated fat, so they can be generously substituted for the high-fat foods that might otherwise be in your diet.

Here are some hints that will help you get even more cholesterol-lowering impact from your use of these foods:

- When selecting breads, choose those that are highest in fiber and lowest in fat content: whole wheat, rye, and French. Breads that use highly refined flours are too low in fiber.

- In the case of rolls, acceptable choices include plain varieties, English and bran muffins, plain bagels, and pita bread. Turn less frequently to bagels made with cheese or eggs, as well as butter rolls, egg bread, doughnuts, croissants, and sweet rolls.

- Plan more lunches and dinners that include spaghetti, macaroni, noodles, rice, wheat, cornmeal, barley, and bulgur (cracked wheat).

- Prepare or buy soups that include high-fiber foods and complex carbohydrates: minestrone, chicken noodle, onion, tomato, split pea, vegetarian vegetable, bouillon, and clam chowder (Manhattan style). But use creamed soups (cream of mushroom, chicken, potato) less often.

- Use low-fat crackers like soda crackers, matzoh, melba toast, and graham crackers. Read the labels on the boxes and avoid those that are made with palm or coconut oil, or use them very sparingly.

♥♥♥♥♥♥♥♥♥♥♥♥♥♥♥♥
DAY 9
♥♥♥♥♥♥♥♥♥♥♥♥♥♥♥♥

Food	SF1 Value	SF2 Value	Cholesterol
Daily Total			

- Make high-fiber cooked and ready-to-eat cereals a daily part of breakfast. Read the nutritional label on the box to select cereals that are low in fat and high in dietary fiber. Avoid those that are made with palm or coconut oil, or use them very sparingly. If you eat cereals with milk, use nonfat or low-fat instead of whole milk.

Substituting two slices of whole wheat bread for one butter croissant reduces the amount of saturated fat you eat by 5.9 grams and the cholesterol by 43 milligrams.

WHAT'S FOR DESSERT?

You don't have to skip dessert to cut out cholesterol, and you don't have to settle for tasteless dishes. When choosing pastries, cut down on commercially prepared treats that are obviously drenched in saturated fats. You can still eat pies and cakes, but choose smaller portions and pick your pastry carefully. There are some delicious options that are quite acceptable—for example, angel food cake, which contains no cholesterol and only trace amounts of fat. Fig bars are relatively low in fat, too, and make another satisfactory choice. You can also bake your own muffins and biscuits at home for snacking, using polyunsaturated oils rather than shortening.

There are many cold desserts you can choose that are ideal for a cholesterol-lowering program. Sherbet is one of them. A cup of orange sherbet has 14 milligrams of cholesterol, and only 13 percent of its calories come from fat. Low-fat and nonfat yogurt make good selections, too. If you must have ice cream on occasion, eat smaller portions and choose one of the low-fat varieties, or try ice milk (in a typical cup of vanilla ice cream, 48 percent of the calories come from fat; that figure drops to 28 percent with ice milk).

Substituting 1/2 cup of gelatin dessert for 1/2 cup of chocolate pudding reduces the amount of saturated fat you eat by 2.4 grams and the cholesterol by 15 milligrams.

♥♥♥♥♥♥♥♥♥♥♥♥♥♥♥
DAY 10
♥♥♥♥♥♥♥♥♥♥♥♥♥♥♥

Food	SF1 Value	SF2 Value	Cholesterol
Daily Total			

CHOOSING SNACK FOODS

The food industry has given us an incredible choice of foods to snack on—even a small market displays hundreds of products, and larger supermarkets stock thousands. The options run all the way from cheese dips and peanuts to soft drinks and potato chips. You can get away with eating almost any of these foods and beverages once in a while, provided your portions are small. But you will have to choose much more carefully if you are a serious "snacker" and you are also serious about getting your cholesterol level down and keeping it there.

Fruits and vegetables are the obvious first choice. You can eat all the fresh apples, pears, and melon you want without having to worry about your cholesterol level. In the process, you will be advancing steadily toward your soluble-fiber goal for the day. Vegetables also provide an almost unlimited source of snack foods that are high in fiber, low in saturated fat or completely free of it, and otherwise extremely nutritious.

Popcorn is another excellent choice, but its effect on your cholesterol level depends on the way you prepare and serve it. Your best option is to pop the kernels in an air popper or use a microwave oven. This leaves considerably less fat on the popcorn than if you use a popper that requires butter or oil.

Finally, if you are going to bathe the popcorn in butter before serving it, you're better off not eating it at all. If you don't like popcorn plain, use a butter substitute.

Tofu is another food item that can be used to prepare tasty snack foods. It has only a moderate amount of fat, yet it can be baked into pies and cheesecakes that feel rich and satisfying. It can also be used in soups and vegetable dishes to replace high-fat dairy products. Tofu (also known as bean curd) is actually a soy cheese made from curdled soy milk. Many supermarkets and health food stores carry tofu in their produce sections.

Substituting one cup of popcorn (air-popped) for one ounce of corn chips reduces the amount of saturated fat you eat by 1.5 grams.

♥♥♥♥♥♥♥♥♥♥♥♥♥♥
DAY 11
♥♥♥♥♥♥♥♥♥♥♥♥♥♥

Food	SF1 Value	SF2 Value	Cholesterol
Daily Total			

CHANGING YOUR SHOPPING HABITS

Now that you are committed to a cholesterol-lowering program, grocery shopping may require a little more of your time and thought. The most important thing you can do is read the label on every food you buy.

Let's look at what is commonly printed in the "Nutritional Information" section of food labels. As an example, we've selected a typical label that might be found on a jar of mayonnaise.

NUTRITION INFORMATION PER SERVING

Serving size	1 tablespoon (14 g)
Servings per container	32
Calories	100
Protein	0
Carbohydrates	0
Fat	11 g
Polyunsaturates	5 g
Saturates	2 g
Cholesterol	5 mg
Sodium	80 mg

Start with the fat content—11 grams per tablespoon. But what does that mean? Is it too high, or just about right? To answer those questions, you need to know the percentage of the calories in mayonnaise that come from fat. And since that information isn't provided on the label, you'll have to calculate it yourself. Once you have that figure in hand, you can decide what kind of effect this particular product is likely to have on your blood cholesterol level.

There's a three-step formula for making this calculation. It may seem a bit complicated, and at first glance you may feel like throwing up your hands in despair. But don't panic. If you will bear with us, you should get the hang of the formula rapidly. Once you do, the calculations will go quickly—and the information you obtain will be invaluable.

♥♥♥♥♥♥♥♥♥♥♥♥♥♥♥
DAY 12
♥♥♥♥♥♥♥♥♥♥♥♥♥♥♥

Food	SF1 Value	SF2 Value	Cholesterol
Daily Total			

1. Multiply the number of grams of fat in one serving by 9 (every gram of fat contains 9 calories, so this calculation will tell you how many *fat* calories there are in each serving).
2. Divide the number you've come up with (the number of fat calories) by the total number of calories in the serving.
3. Finally, take the number you've arrived at in step 2 and multiply by 100 to convert it to a percentage (an easy way to do that is simply to move the decimal point two digits to the right). Now you have the information you're after: the percentage of calories that come from fat.

Referring back to our sample mayonnaise label, you would multiply 11 grams (the number of grams of fat in a single serving) by 9 (the number of calories in each gram of fat), and the answer is 99. Divide that by 100 (the total number of calories in a single serving) and the result is .99. Then multiply that figure by 100 to convert it to a percentage.

This mathematical exercise (which looks more difficult than it really is) will show you that 99 percent of all the calories in mayonnaise are in the form of fat. That is disturbingly high when you are being so careful to keep your total dietary fat intake to less than 30 percent of your caloric intake. The label also reveals another important piece of information—in this particular product, there is 2.5 times more polyunsaturated fat than saturated fat. That is a good sign, since it is the saturated fats in particular that you are trying to keep to an absolute minimum. However, you are still going to get two grams of saturated fat for every tablespoon of mayonnaise you consume.

Substituting one ounce of part-skim mozzarella cheese for one ounce of cheddar reduces the amount of saturated fat you eat by 2.9 grams and the cholesterol by 9 milligrams.

♥♥♥♥♥♥♥♥♥♥♥♥♥♥♥
DAY 13
♥♥♥♥♥♥♥♥♥♥♥♥♥♥♥

Food	SF1 Value	SF2 Value	Cholesterol
Daily Total			

READING THE LIST OF INGREDIENTS

On most food labels you will find a list that contains every ingredient used in the manufacture or processing of the product. According to government regulations, the ingredients must be listed in descending order by weight—that is, the ingredient listed first is present in the greatest amount, and the last ingredient in the smallest quantity. For example, the mayonnaise label reads:

> INGREDIENTS: Soybean oil, partially hydrogenated soybean oil, whole eggs, water, vinegar, egg yolks, sugar, salt, lemon juice, natural flavors, and disodium EDTA added to protect flavor.

When reading labels, you have to be especially alert for the names of saturated fats, such as coconut oil, palm oil, butter, cream, beef fat, and lard. If they appear anywhere near the top of the list, you should try to find a similar food that has been made with unsaturated oils.

Look also for the presence of whole eggs or egg yolks (the whites are no problem) in baked or processed foods. Most of the eggs produced in the United States are used in such foods. If you don't read the labels, you could end up eating far more cholesterol because of these eggs than you imagined possible.

Unfortunately, some food labels are rather deceptive. For instance, a label that says only "contains vegetable oil," could be loaded with an oil that is very high in saturated fat. The best strategy is to shy away from products that are so vague about their contents, and seek out those that are not afraid to provide specific information.

Substituting one tablespoon of imitation mayonnaise for one tablespoon of real mayonnaise reduces the amount of saturated fat you eat by 1.1 grams and the cholesterol by 4 milligrams.

▼▼▼▼▼▼▼▼▼▼▼▼▼▼▼▼
DAY 14
▼▼▼▼▼▼▼▼▼▼▼▼▼▼▼▼

Food	SF1 Value	SF2 Value	Cholesterol
Daily Total			

WHEN IS A PRODUCT REALLY "97% FAT FREE"?

Be wary when a product claims to contain "only 3% fat" or to be "97% fat free." (You will frequently find this kind of statement on cold cuts such as sliced ham or salami.) That usually means that 3 percent of the product *by weight* is fat. But weight isn't the crucial factor—calories are. One popular "97% fat free" meat product actually gets 36 percent of its calories from fat. Another, promoted as "94% fat free," gets 51 percent of its calories from fat. Though the manufacturers of these products are correct in a technical sense, neither product qualifies as a low-fat food. You have to control your intake of such products carefully.

You can get around this problem by purchasing only products that give you the exact amount of fat content in grams. That's a figure you can count on. This approach, however, will significantly restrict your choices, because relatively few manufacturers provide these details on their labels. But it's worth living with that restriction in order to get your blood cholesterol level down. If you want to know how much *saturated* fat is in the product, and the label doesn't contain that information, check the SF1 Food Lists for it. You will find the saturated fat content for most commonly eaten foods.

Substituting 3 1/2 ounces of cured ham steak for 3 1/2 ounces of fried bacon reduces the amount of saturated fat you eat by 16 grams and the cholesterol by 40 milligrams.

♥♥♥♥♥♥♥♥♥♥♥♥♥♥♥
DAY 15
♥♥♥♥♥♥♥♥♥♥♥♥♥♥♥

Food	SF1 Value	SF2 Value	Cholesterol
Daily Total			

BE WARY ABOUT "NO-CHOLESTEROL" LABELS

Obviously, the less cholesterol a food product has, the better. But even the words "no cholesterol" or "cholesterol-free" on a label are no guarantee that the food is appropriate for someone on a cholesterol-lowering diet. Cholesterol-free foods—even those of vegetable origin—can still contain large amounts of saturated fats, and that may cause your cholesterol level to go up (the best examples of this are foods that use palm or coconut oil or other highly saturated vegetable oils).

You will find these "no cholesterol" labels on margarines, crackers, cereals, mayonnaise, potato chips, and many other foods. But you can't rely only on this claim in deciding what particular product or brand to buy. Read the rest of the label carefully to be sure that this isn't just a deceptive claim for a product that is high in saturated fat.

Substituting one fluid ounce of coconut oil for one fluid ounce of corn oil *increases* the amount of saturated fat you eat by 20.2 grams (there is no cholesterol in either oil). Although processed foods made with coconut oil can legitimately claim that they contain no cholesterol, their saturated-fat content is much higher than that of similar foods made with other vegetable oils.

♥♥♥♥♥♥♥♥♥♥♥♥♥♥♥
DAY 16
♥♥♥♥♥♥♥♥♥♥♥♥♥♥♥

Food	SF1 Value	SF2 Value	Cholesterol
Daily Total			

USING YOUR FAVORITE RECIPES

You do not have to give up your favorite dishes just because you're try-ing to lower your cholesterol level, but you may have to make a few modifications in the basic recipes. Use the following list as a guide to ingredient exchanges that will help you eliminate saturated fat and cho-lesterol. These exchanges may alter the texture and taste of the dishes slightly, but with a little experimentation you can convert your recipes to a healthier state without sacrificing any of their taste or pleasure.

In place of	Use
whole milk	skim milk
sour cream	nonfat yogurt
butter	margarine
cheese	hoop, sapsago cheese
whole egg	egg whites
ice cream	frozen yogurt
shortening	unsaturated vegetable oil
white flour	whole wheat flour

Substituting 2 ounces of low-fat plain yogurt for 2 ounces of sour cream reduces the amount of saturated fat you eat by 5.9 grams and the cholesterol by 17 milligrams.

♥♥♥♥♥♥♥♥♥♥♥♥♥♥♥
DAY 17
♥♥♥♥♥♥♥♥♥♥♥♥♥♥♥

Food	SF1 Value	SF2 Value	Cholesterol
Daily Total			

CHOOSING THE BEST OILS

All oils are not born equal—not even vegetable oils. They vary considerably in their amount of saturated and polyunsaturated fats and, therefore, in their effect on your blood cholesterol level. To lower your level, you need to limit your use of oils to those that are high in polyunsaturated fats and low in saturated fats. The ones you should use (in order of decreasing amounts of polyunsaturated fats) are safflower, corn, soybean, cottonseed, sunflower, and canola. At the opposite end of the spectrum are the ones to avoid or to consume in small quantities: coconut, palm, and palm kernel oils, which are all high in saturated fat. The latter group of fats are frequently found in products such as bakery goods, microwave popcorn, nondairy creamers, and processed foods.

When choosing dressings for your salads, you'll want to cut down on blue cheese, Roquefort, and any other dressings made with cheese or sour cream. As an alternative, prepare your own salad dressing with safflower, sunflower, or corn oil, or use a little lemon and vinegar to add flavor and tang to the dish.

One final reminder. Even though polyunsaturated fats and oils are clearly preferable to saturated fats, you shouldn't overdo your intake of them, either.

Substituting one tablespoon of safflower oil for one tablespoon of butter in your cooking reduces the amount of saturated fat you eat by 5.9 grams and the cholesterol by 31 milligrams.

♥♥♥♥♥♥♥♥♥♥♥♥♥♥♥
DAY 18
♥♥♥♥♥♥♥♥♥♥♥♥♥♥♥

Food	SF1 Value	SF2 Value	Cholesterol
Daily Total			

DINING OUT

When you dine at a restaurant, someone else is in charge in the kitchen, but that doesn't mean you have to give up control of what you eat. Don't be bashful about telling your waiter or waitress that you are on a cholesterol-lowering program and asking for exactly the dishes you want. Most chefs are eager to please their customers, and willing to prepare tempting dishes that meet their health requirements. Here are some more tips for staying on a cholesterol-lowering program while enjoying a meal out.

- Choose the same healthy foods you would eat at home, avoiding the high-fat cuts of beef and pork. If you order chicken or turkey, ask the chef to remove the skin before it is cooked.

- Don't be reluctant to ask that your dish be prepared in a different manner than the way it is described on the menu. A good chef will be happy to broil, bake, or poach a fish for you—even though the menu describes it as swimming in Hollandaise sauce.

- Ask that all sauces be served on the side. That allows you to taste the sauce without having to eat as much. If the food is inadvertently sent out covered with sauce, send it right back and ask for a different portion.

- If you get swept along with others to a steak house, don't despair. Order a small cut, and take home whatever is left over for someone else to eat.

- Order a vegetable plate, even if you don't see one on the menu. Every restaurant is prepared to make such a dish on a moment's notice, especially if you explain why it's important to you. A good chef will go out of the way to make your vegetables a memorable meal.

- Choose seafood salads if they're available, but go easy on the shrimp; unless you cover the seafood in cream-based sauces or oil, you are practically guaranteed a meal low in saturated fat.

♥♥♥♥♥♥♥♥♥♥♥♥♥♥
DAY 19
♥♥♥♥♥♥♥♥♥♥♥♥♥♥

Food	SF1 Value	SF2 Value	Cholesterol
Daily Total			

- At salad bars, help yourself to generous portions of beans, cauliflower, celery, radishes, broccoli, and other fresh vegetables. Limit your portions of coleslaw, eggs, avocados, cheese, olives, croutons, marinated vegetables (because of the oil in which they're prepared), and salad dressing.

- If bread is served, ask for whole wheat, sour dough, or rye, rather than butter rolls and croissants. If you use butter or margarine, do so sparingly.

- For breakfast, you can't go wrong with hot cereal, unless you melt a lot of butter on top of it. Cold cereals offer a perfect start to a low-fat, low-cholesterol day, especially if you fill your bowl with nonfat (skim) milk.

- When traveling long distances by plane, call the airline ahead of time and request a low-cholesterol meal. In addition to being good for you, these special meals are often more tasty and attractive than the regular airline fare.

Substituting 7 ounces of white turkey meat (without skin) for 7 ounces of spare ribs reduces the amount of saturated fat you eat by 22.8 grams and the cholesterol by 65 milligrams.

♥♥♥♥♥♥♥♥♥♥♥♥♥♥
DAY 20
♥♥♥♥♥♥♥♥♥♥♥♥♥♥

Food	SF1 Value	SF2 Value	Cholesterol
Daily Total			

EATING ETHNIC FOODS OUT

French restaurants—notorious for their high-fat sauces—need not be avoided, but you will have to be selective in choosing dishes, and you should ask if the sauces can be served on the side. If you must taste the organ meats or pâté, order a small portion and share it with everyone at the table.

Chinese and Japanese restaurants typically offer many low-fat, low-cholesterol options. If you have a choice, pick steamed or stir-fried chicken or fish and rice instead of deep-fried dishes such as tempura or pork-fried rice. Fortune cookies are a good choice for a low-fat dessert; almond cookies are less desirable.

Eating Italian food out is no problem either, if you eat the meatless pasta dishes, such as spaghetti with tomato or marinara sauce. If you sprinkle Parmesan cheese on your pasta, do so sparingly. If you choose meat, poultry, or fish, order a sauce that is low in fat.

In Mexican restaurants, low-fat, low-cholesterol ingredients are often turned into high-fat dishes that are loaded with calories. Beware of chips soaked with oil and refried beans cooked with lard. Steer away from the deep-fried chile rellenos stuffed with cheese and toward the chicken and fish dishes.

Substituting lemon juice for four tablespoons of Hollandaise sauce reduces the amount of saturated fat you eat by 7 grams and the cholesterol by 30 milligrams.

♥♥♥♥♥♥♥♥♥♥♥♥♥♥♥
DAY 21
♥♥♥♥♥♥♥♥♥♥♥♥♥♥♥

Food	SF1 Value	SF2 Value	Cholesterol
Daily Total			

SHOULD YOU AVOID FAST FOOD?

Though "fast food" restaurants are notorious for their high-fat menus, almost all of these restaurants now offer selections that are perfectly compatible with a cholesterol-lowering program. So don't blame the restaurant industry if you pick the wrong dish or patronize a restaurant that doesn't offer the foods you should be eating.

Here are some points to keep in mind when eating in a fast-food restaurant.

- As much as possible, try to avoid fried foods, particularly if they are fried in coconut oil or beef fat (ask the restaurant manager what kind of oil is being used). Some restaurants are using highly saturated fats for cooking, but many chains—responding to consumer pressure for healthier foods—are switching to polyunsaturated vegetable oils for food preparation.
- Fill your plate at the salad bar, but try to avoid the high-fat dressings and be sparing in your consumption of cheese, eggs, bacon, and the like.
- If you order a baked potato, don't let them bury it in butter, sour cream, or cheese, all of which can turn this low-fat dish into a high-fat, high-cholesterol nightmare.
- If you are in the mood for a hamburger, pick the smallest one on the menu, and order it without cheese or mayonnaise.
- Top your pizzas with vegetables. Though pepperoni and sausage do add flavor, they also significantly increase the amount of saturated fat and cholesterol in each slice.

Substituting 8 ounces of nonfat milk for a 10-ounce chocolate milk shake reduces the amount of saturated fat you eat by 6.2 grams and the cholesterol by 33 milligrams.

♥♥♥♥♥♥♥♥♥♥♥♥♥♥
DAY 22
♥♥♥♥♥♥♥♥♥♥♥♥♥♥

Food	SF1 Value	SF2 Value	Cholesterol
Daily Total			

COFFEE AND CHOLESTEROL

In a highly publicized study published in 1983, Norwegian researchers reported that drinking coffee caused elevated blood cholesterol and triglyceride levels in healthy men and women. Men who consumed from one to four cups of coffee per day had an average total cholesterol level of 228, compared to 215 for those who drank less than a cup a day, and 241 for those who consumed more than eight cups. This gave credence to the idea that coffee-drinking and cholesterol were related. However, since subsequent investigations by others reached contradictory conclusions, you don't need to stop drinking coffee to lower your blood cholesterol. Bear in mind, however, that coffee whiteners *can* cause problems. Cream is high in saturated fat, as are nondairy whiteners that contain coconut oil.

Substituting one cup of black coffee for one cup of flavored instant mocha coffee reduces the amount of saturated fat you eat by 2.4 grams.

♥♥♥♥♥♥♥♥♥♥♥♥♥♥♥
DAY 23
♥♥♥♥♥♥♥♥♥♥♥♥♥♥♥

Food	SF1 Value	SF2 Value	Cholesterol
Daily Total			

WHAT ABOUT GARLIC?

Garlic may do more than just create an offensive odor that could hamper your social life. Some research has found that garlic extracts can positively influence blood cholesterol levels. For instance, when researchers at Tulane University conducted a 12-week study comparing the effects of garlic tablets (90 mg a day) with placebos, they discovered that garlic reduced average blood cholesterol levels from 262 to 247. LDL cholesterol dropped 11 percent, but there was no significant change in HDL cholesterol. A so-called "meta-analysis" evaluating five studies of garlic, reported by New York Medical College researchers in 1993, concluded that garlic (about 1/2 to 1 clove per day) decreased total cholesterol levels by about 9 percent.

What's the bottom line? Although you can use garlic as one of your weapons against high blood cholesterol levels, the other strategies in this book should still receive your top priority.

HOT DOGS: SOME FRANK INFORMATION

A backyard barbecue or a baseball game just would not be the same without a hot dog, but there's a price to pay for this all-American meal. In a typical beef frankfurter, about 82 percent of the calories come from fat, and more than 40 percent of these fat calories are saturated. Turkey hot dogs—marketed as a healthier substitute for beef and pork franks—work out a little better, because they have fewer calories (about 115 compared to 160 in a beef frank). Still, 70 percent of these calories come from fat, and 33 percent of the fat calories are saturated. Chicken hot dogs are a somewhat better choice; although 68 percent of their calories come from fat, only about 28 percent of these fat calories are saturated.

Substituting two turkey frankfurters for two beef frankfurters reduces the amount of saturated fat you eat by 6.4 grams and increases the amount of cholesterol by 20 milligrams.

♥♥♥♥♥♥♥♥♥♥♥♥♥♥
DAY 24
♥♥♥♥♥♥♥♥♥♥♥♥♥♥

Food	SF1 Value	SF2 Value	Cholesterol
Daily Total			

STICKING WITH YOUR EXERCISE PROGRAM

You can't raise your HDL level with just an occasional day of vigorous exercise. That takes regular physical activity. But everyone has days when he or she would rather not exercise, and there are a million excuses you can find to get out of it: the weather, a busy schedule, a trip—the list goes on and on. If you let those excuses keep you inactive for any extended period of time, you quickly lose whatever gains you've achieved with exercise in the past. Here's what you can do to keep that from happening.

- Schedule your exercise period just as you would any other daily activity. Literally write an appointment for exercise into your datebook or calendar each day, just as you would for any important appointment (preferably at the same time each day). If exercise becomes an important part of your routine, you are more likely to stick with it.

- To avoid boredom, change your walking (or running) route often. Explore different parts of your neighborhood, or drive to a starting point elsewhere and explore new scenery.

- Find an exercise partner who agrees to join you regularly. On the days when you just don't feel like working out, your partner may give you the extra push you need to get moving. Also, when exercise turns into a social event, it becomes more enjoyable.

Substituting one slice of cheese pizza (1/8 of a 15" pizza) for quiche lorraine (1/8 of an 8" pie) reduces the amount of saturated fat you eat by 19.1 grams and the cholesterol by 229 milligrams.

♥♥♥♥♥♥♥♥♥♥♥♥♥♥♥♥
DAY 25
♥♥♥♥♥♥♥♥♥♥♥♥♥♥♥♥

Food	SF1 Value	SF2 Value	Cholesterol
Daily Total			

CHOOSING CHICKEN AND TURKEY

Because of increasing interest in cholesterol, the popularity of poultry is on the rise, and there is good reason for it. Poultry tends to be lower in total fat, saturated fat, cholesterol, and calories than most popular cuts of beef and pork. However, not all poultry was created equal. So careful selections in this category can make an even greater difference. Here are some facts you can use when shopping for poultry.

- In general, turkey and chicken have less fat than other types of poultry, such as duck and goose.
- White poultry meat has about half the fat of dark meat. Breast meat is particularly lean (skinless turkey breast is nearly fat-free, although it does contain cholesterol). Small, younger chickens (broilers, fryers) are leaner than larger, older ones.
- Broiling, baking, or roasting are your best options for cooking poultry. You can also poach it in vegetable juice or broth. If you fry poultry—particularly if the skin is left on—the amounts of fat and calories soar—a real problem especially if there is much saturated fat in the oil or shortening you use.

Substituting 3 1/2 ounces of light skinless turkey for 3 1/2 ounces of roasted duck (flesh only) reduces the amount of saturated fat you eat by 3.8 grams and the cholesterol by 3 milligrams.

♥♥♥♥♥♥♥♥♥♥♥♥♥♥
DAY 26
♥♥♥♥♥♥♥♥♥♥♥♥♥♥

Food	SF1 Value	SF2 Value	Cholesterol
Daily Total			

MORE ABOUT OATS, BEANS, AND BLACK-EYED PEAS

In the discussion of the benefits of fiber in Chapter Nine, oat bran, beans, and black-eyed peas were singled out as foods rich in soluble fiber and easy to incorporate into your meals. In addition to the suggestions on page 118, there are other ways of making these foods a regular part of your diet. The following hints will be helpful when choosing and cooking these health-promoting foods.

- Use many different varieties of beans and legumes— each has its own unique taste and consistency. Cook them as many different ways as you can; each variation adds interest and attraction to a group of foods that deserve it.

- Use beans and legumes as condiments. Add them to soups and stews and sprinkle them on salads. Use beans to replace beef in your recipes (this works especially well for Mexican dishes). This not only increases the amount of soluble fiber in the dish but adds to its overall nutritional value.

- When you purchase beans in cans, read the labels carefully to be sure that a lot of salt has not been added to them.

- Presoak the beans for several hours before cooking. Then drain them and add fresh water before you cook them. This eliminates some of the carbohydrates that can cause excess gas. You can also reduce the problem of flatulence by not eating other gaseous foods (such as cabbage) at the same time.

Substituting 1/2 cup of cooked kidney beans for 1/2 cup of cooked broccoli will increase the amount of soluble fiber you eat by 2.0 grams.

♥♥♥♥♥♥♥♥♥♥♥♥♥♥♥
DAY 27
♥♥♥♥♥♥♥♥♥♥♥♥♥♥♥

Food	SF1 Value	SF2 Value	Cholesterol
Daily Total			

SURVIVING A DINNER PARTY

Dinner parties in other people's homes pose more difficult problems when you're on a cholesterol-lowering program—but not impossible ones. The following hints may help you control your fat and fiber intake without ruffling the feathers of any friends. By the way, if being a good guest causes you to miss your SF goals for a day, don't panic. One research study shows that deviating from a low-fat diet occasionally—once every week or two—won't raise your blood cholesterol level significantly if you really stick to the plan the rest of the time.

- Let your host or hostess know a few days before the party that you are trying to stay on a low-fat, cholesterol-lowering diet. Make sure the planned menu is something you can eat without problems, or volunteer to bring a special dish for yourself.

- If you arrive at a party and you are not happy with the main course, ask for a tiny portion and fill the rest of your plate with salad and vegetables. Go light on the salad dressing and avoid butter on the vegetables, and you won't have to feel guilty about eating a little of the main dish.

- Go easy on the appetizers, especially those that are fried or made with high-fat cheeses or sour cream. Just a few minutes of careless snacking can undo all your later good efforts at dinner.

- No matter what is being served to others, request fruit for your dessert. This shouldn't inconvenience your hosts at all, it protects you, and it sets an excellent example for everyone else at the table.

Substituting four ounces of low-fat (1%) cottage cheese for four ounces of creamed cottage cheese reduces the amount of saturated fat you eat by 2.5 grams and the cholesterol by 12 milligrams.

♥♥♥♥♥♥♥♥♥♥♥♥♥♥♥
DAY 28
♥♥♥♥♥♥♥♥♥♥♥♥♥♥♥

Food	SF1 Value	SF2 Value	Cholesterol
Daily Total			

MAKING THE BEST CHOICES OF NUTS

Nuts are a favorite snack food for many Americans. Not only do people eat them by the handful, but they are commonly found mixed into many other types of foods, ranging from cereals (such as granola) to peanut butter.

At first glance, nuts might seem to be a good choice for snacking. After all, most of them have a relatively low saturated-fat content. A 1 oz. serving of almonds, for instance, contains 1.4 grams of saturated fat; that means that less than 8 percent of its calories come from saturated fat. Many other types of nuts fare just as well. Pecans have 1.5 grams of saturated fat in a 1 oz. serving, and saturated fats make up about 7 percent of their calories.

But as good as this may sound, it can be a little misleading. Most nuts, in fact, contain high levels of *total* fat and thus are high in calories as well. Almonds have 167 calories in each 1 oz. serving, and 80 percent of these calories are from fat! Pecans have 187 calories in the same size serving, and 89 percent come from fat. Thus, particularly if you are watching your weight, you need to limit the amount of nuts you incorporate into your diet.

Incidentally, one type of nut—European chestnuts—is an exception to this rule. Chestnuts are not only low in saturated fat (0.2 gram for every ounce), but low in total fat and thus not as high in calories (105 calories per ounce) as other types of nuts. Only 9 percent of the calories in chestnuts come from fat.

Substituting one ounce of European chestnuts for an equal portion of macadamia nuts reduces the amount of saturated fat you eat by 2.9 grams. Neither variety of nut contains any cholesterol.

♥♥♥♥♥♥♥♥♥♥♥♥♥♥♥
DAY 29
♥♥♥♥♥♥♥♥♥♥♥♥♥♥♥

Food	SF1 Value	SF2 Value	Cholesterol
Daily Total			

WHERE TO GET ADDITIONAL HELP

By now, you have the information and tools you need to implement the dietary program recommended in this book. Even so, from time to time, you may feel that you need some additional help.

If that happens, turn to your doctor's office. Your physician or a qualified person on the office staff can answer diet-related questions you may have, and help you through any troublesome areas. In some cases, your doctor might recommend that you see a registered dietician or qualified nutritionist for some additional guidance. These health professionals can help identify problems with your eating behavior, and can give you some specialized advice on shopping for and preparing cholesterol-lowering foods. You can also locate a dietician through a local hospital, or by contacting the state or district office of the American Dietetic Association.

Particularly if your blood cholesterol level has not decreased substantially after following this program for a month or two, a registered dietician may be able to troubleshoot for you. He or she can analyze your eating habits at home and in restaurants, pinpointing problems and making recommendations to get you back on track. Your own personal situation—for instance, your health difficulties, your lifestyle, or your family circumstances—can be taken into account during this type of one-on-one consultation.

♥♥♥♥♥♥♥♥♥♥♥♥♥♥♥
DAY 30
♥♥♥♥♥♥♥♥♥♥♥♥♥♥♥

Food	SF1 Value	SF2 Value	Cholesterol
Daily Total			

12

♥ ♥ ♥ ♥

EVALUATING YOUR PROGRESS

Since high blood cholesterol itself causes no symptoms, you will have no way of knowing how your body is responding to this program unless your blood cholesterol level is remeasured. The time for that measurement depends to some extent on how high your reading was before you started this program. If your blood cholesterol level was 200 to 239 and you had no other risk factors that placed you in the "high-risk" group, no further testing is necessary for a year (according to guidelines established by the National Cholesterol Education Program). However, you and your doctor may choose to repeat the cholesterol measurement earlier if you are curious about the results of your cholesterol-lowering efforts. You should discuss ahead of time what cholesterol level would make you feel you had achieved success, and what you should do if the blood test shows that you have not reached this goal.

If your cholesterol level before you start is 240 or over, or if you have other factors that place you at risk for heart disease, the NCEP guidelines recommend that your total blood cholesterol be remeasured four to six weeks after you adopt a better eating pattern and again at three months.

This will enable you and your physician to determine how well your body is responding to the dietary therapy. Within this category, a dietary program is considered to have achieved its *minimal* goal if the total blood cholesterol has declined to less than 240 in people without coronary heart disease or two other risk factors, and less than 200 in people who have coronary heart disease or two other risk factors. (Note: These are *minimal* goals; lower levels are considered even more desirable.)

You and your doctor may choose a different end-point as the level that you would consider acceptable. As discussed in Chapter Six, it is also important to remember that errors can occur in measuring your blood cholesterol. If a repeat blood test fails to show any reduction in your cholesterol level, your doctor may wish to perform the test again before concluding that your body has really not responded to dietary measures.

There are several reasons why your body might not respond adequately to a cholesterol-lowering diet:

1. If your original blood cholesterol level was extremely high, you may be able to lower your cholesterol to some degree, but not enough to reach an acceptable level of risk.

2. You may be one of those persons whose body is biologically resistant to dietary changes (less than 5 percent of people with high blood cholesterol fall into this category). In that case, you may need to adopt a diet that is even lower in saturated fat and cholesterol than the one you have been following, or you may be so biologically resistant that you will not be able to achieve your goal with *any* diet, no matter how strict. (Other strategies, particularly drug therapy, may be appropriate in the latter case.)

3. You may not have been following the diet as closely as you thought you were, and you may need dietary counseling and a little more practice to get it right.

If you did not reach your goal, there are several possible options available to you. Discuss each of the following with your doctor to see which is most appropriate in your particular case:

1. Continue the same diet for three more months, checking your cholesterol level in about four weeks and once again at the end of three months to see if it responds to this therapy.

2. Switch to the Step Two Diet (see below) for three months, checking your cholesterol level in four weeks and again at the end of three months.

3. Begin drug therapy in *addition* to continuing your diet (either the original diet or the Step Two Diet). This approach may be appropriate if your original cholesterol level was so high that your doctor believes that diet alone will not lower it to an acceptable level.

THE STEP TWO DIET

The Step Two Diet differs from the diet recommended in Chapters Eight, Nine, and Ten. The amount of saturated fat consumed is limited to less than 7 percent of the total caloric intake each day (compared to 10 percent), and the amount of dietary cholesterol is kept under 200 milligrams per day (compared to 300).

The amount of soluble fiber eaten each day on the Step Two Diet remains the same as on the original program, so your SF2 number remains the same. However, the amount of saturated fat you are allowed drops by 30 percent, so you will need a new SF1 number to guide your decisions about saturated fat.

To identify your new SF1 number for the Step Two Diet, use the chart that follows. Find the point at which your ideal weight intersects with your activity level; that figure is now your SF1 number. Next, review the SF1 food charts on pages 77–86, and notice which foods you may now have to eat less frequently or in smaller portions to achieve your new daily goal. Remember, your SF1 food totals each day should not exceed your new SF1 number.

Chart 21

PERSONAL SF1 NUMBERS FOR STEP TWO DIET: MEN

Desirable Weight	Activity Level		
	Inactive	Moderately Active	Very Active
90	10	11	11
100	11	12	12
110	12	13	14
120	13	14	15
130	14	15	16
140	15	16	17
150	16	18	19
160	17	19	20
170	19	20	21
180	20	21	22
190	21	22	24
200	22	23	25
210	23	25	26
220	24	26	27

PERSONAL SF1 NUMBERS FOR STEP TWO DIET: WOMEN

Desirable Weight	Activity Level		
	Inactive	Moderately Active	Very Active
90	9	9	10
100	10	11	11
110	11	12	12
120	12	13	13
130	13	14	15
140	14	15	16
150	15	16	17
160	16	17	18
170	17	18	19
180	18	19	20
190	19	20	21
200	20	21	22
210	21	22	24
220	22	23	25

OTHER WAYS TO MEASURE PROGRESS

While your primary objective in following this program is to lower your blood cholesterol level, you may be gaining some other benefits, too. This is a good time to take stock of any advantages your new diet and lifestyle are providing. The more benefits you recognize, the more you will enjoy the process and the more likely you will be to maintain your new health habits.

Are you enjoying meals more? Do you like the variety of foods and textures your new diet is bringing you? Do you like the new and varied tastes you are experiencing? Do you feel better about yourself after eating a meal that you know is good for you? Take note of every pleasure, because this will reinforce your healthier eating habits and help make them a lifetime pattern.

Have you lost any weight? This happens frequently to people who switch to foods that are low in saturated fat (and therefore lower in total fat and total calories) and who start eating more high-fiber foods (which tend, by their very nature, to be low in calories and more filling).

Do you feel more fit? Are you looking better? Are you coughing less? If you have been exercising more often and you have given up smoking, your answer to all of these questions will probably be "yes." Don't take these wonderful sensations for granted. Make a point of thinking about them. Each time you do, you will be rewarded even more for your new commitment to health.

Remember that it takes years of this healthy lifestyle for you to earn the fullest rewards. A lifelong pattern of low-fat, high-fiber eating increases your chance of longevity and enhances the quality of your life, while at the same time lowering your risk of coronary heart disease. Whatever the results of your cholesterol tests and the other measures of your well-being at this time, make a commitment to this way of eating and living for the rest of your life. That's how long you'll be enjoying the benefits.

13

♥　♥　♥　♥

MEDICAL THERAPIES
When Diet and Exercise
Aren't Enough

Most people can reduce their blood cholesterol levels and their risk of coronary heart disease to acceptable levels with dietary measures alone. However, some individuals—no matter how closely they adhere to a cholesterol-lowering diet—are unable to lower their levels far enough. Generally, these people have hereditary problems that cause their livers to manufacture excess cholesterol, and that interfere with the normal mechanisms for taking cholesterol out of the blood. For these individuals, prescription medications may be an important second step—not an alternative to a cholesterol-lowering diet but an addition to it.

Several drugs have been available for this purpose for years, and some new medicines have come on the market more recently. The drugs vary in the way they cause cholesterol levels to fall and in the size of the decrease they produce, so the decision about which drug to use must be tailored by a physician to meet the particular needs of each patient. Also, the drugs differ significantly in terms of their side effects, so a drug that is well tolerated by one person may be unacceptable for another.

None of the drugs is a cure for high blood cholesterol. (There is no cure at this time—not even with diet—in spite of some claims to the contrary.) Like dietary measures, which *control* (not cure) blood cholesterol levels only as long as they are followed, drugs *control* cholesterol levels only as long as they are taken. Therefore, the decision to start on a drug must be thought of as a commitment to long-term treatment with medication—in some cases, a lifelong commitment.

Some of these medications are capable of producing dramatic drops in blood cholesterol levels—up to 40 percent under certain circumstances. But the benefits of such exciting results must be weighed against (*a*) the possibility that adverse side effects will occur and (*b*) the cost of the drugs, which can be very significant. For these reasons, cholesterol-lowering drugs are generally recommended only when dietary measures have failed to produce an adequate response. The exception to this rule is when a person's initial cholesterol level is so high—for example, 400 or 500, as in the case of some people with hereditary disorders—that a physician might recommend starting both dietary measures *and* drugs at the same time.

There is no absolute blood cholesterol level above or below which drugs should or should not be used. However, the National Cholesterol Education Program has established some guidelines that can help determine when to consider drug therapy. These NCEP guidelines are based on the amount of LDL cholesterol in the blood, not on the total blood cholesterol, so a lipid profile that specifically measures LDL should be done before a person is started on cholesterol-lowering medications.

According to the NCEP, if a person has definite coronary heart disease (CHD)—or two risk factors for CHD in addition to high blood cholesterol (one of which can be the male sex)—drug therapy should be considered when a dietary program has failed to bring the LDL cholesterol level down to 159 or below. (In most people, this would be equivalent to a total blood cholesterol level of about 240 to 250.) For people who do *not* have either definite CHD or two additional risk factors for it, the NCEP recommends that drug therapy be considered if a dietary plan fails to bring the LDL cholesterol level down to 189 or below. (This corresponds in most people to a total blood cholesterol of about 280 to 300.) Different LDL cholesterol levels for starting drug therapy (160 vs. 190) have been designated for the two groups since the first set of circumstances is considered to pose more immediate risk for a heart attack than the second.

The NCEP emphasizes that these are only guidelines—not rules to be applied across the board. For example, many physicians would choose to start medications at lower blood cholesterol levels than these in a very young person, while letting an individual who is seventy or eighty go without medications at all. In the final analysis, the decision about whether or not to start drug therapy is one that must be decided on an individual basis. If your blood cholesterol level remains high in spite of dietary measures, your doctor will review with you the potential benefits and disadvantages of drug therapy, and together you can make the decision that is best for your particular circumstances.

There is one point about drug therapy that is appropriate for everyone and cannot be overemphasized—this treatment should not be used as a substitute for a cholesterol-lowering diet but as a *supplement* to it, and only when dietary therapy is ineffective at reaching an acceptable cholesterol level. One cannot justify taking the additional risk of drug therapy when diet alone would achieve the same results. Besides, drugs produce better results when used in combination with a low-fat, low-cholesterol diet.

Furthermore, the NCEP's expert panel recommends that cholesterol-lowering diets be given enough time to work before drugs are started. The panel advises six months of intensive dietary therapy before medications are prescribed, except in people with very severe elevations of LDL cholesterol (over 225, which corresponds to a total blood cholesterol of about 300 or more) or with definite CHD. However, these guidelines are based in part on the belief that it takes several months before people are able to change their dietary habits fully. As you learned earlier, it takes nowhere near that long to reach the lowest blood cholesterol level that dietary changes can produce, so your own physician may recommend drug therapy much earlier if he or she is convinced that you have meticulously followed the cholesterol-lowering dietary plan described in this book.

Finally, the NCEP recommends that during the first few months of drug therapy, the patient's response to medication should be monitored by repeating the LDL measurements at regular intervals. Once a stable level is reached, the less expensive total blood cholesterol measurement can be used, since it tends to parallel the LDL figures (Remember, LDL cholesterol accounts for 60 to 70 percent of the total blood cholesterol.)

WHAT DRUGS ARE AVAILABLE?

Your doctor has several options to choose from when selecting cholesterol-lowering drugs. There are now several major types of drugs, and they lower blood cholesterol levels in somewhat different ways. The material that follows will provide you with enough information about the various drugs to prepare you to discuss them with your doctor. Remember, no two people are alike, so your particular circumstances might make one drug more desirable than another.

Nicotinic Acid (Niacin)

Nicotinic acid, a member of the "B" vitamin group (B3), has been used by physicians for many years to lower blood cholesterol levels. It produces this effect by decreasing production of very low density lipoproteins (VLDL), which in turn results in the creation of less LDL cholesterol. In most studies, nicotinic acid has reduced LDL cholesterol levels 15 to 30 percent and *increased* HDL levels 20 percent or more in some patients—and this has resulted in real health benefits. In one study, when survivors of heart attacks received nicotinic acid, they suffered 21 percent fewer repeat nonfatal heart attacks than patients who did not, and their long-term survival rate was 11 percent better than that of the group not taking the vitamin.

Nicotinic acid (also called "niacin") must be used in very high doses to achieve these positive effects—doses that create a real risk of toxicity and produce a high incidence of discomforting side effects. At these dosage levels, it is more appropriate to think of nicotinic acid as a powerful drug that should be used under the supervision of a physician rather than as a harmless vitamin. Severe flushing of the skin ("hot flashes" is the way many people describe it) is probably the best-known adverse effect, occurring one to two hours after the preparation is ingested. This flushing can be so unpleasant that many people discontinue using nicotinic acid altogether. However, there is no danger associated with this symptom, and the redness of the skin disappears on its own, leaving no aftereffects.

Flushing may be less likely to occur if nicotinic acid is started at a very low dosage and built up gradually to higher levels. It may also help to take the drug with meals and to avoid drinking alcohol or hot beverages at the same time. Some studies suggest that the flushing can be minimized if one takes an aspirin tablet thirty minutes before each dose of nicotinic acid. The use of timed-release nicotinic acid preparations may also prevent or minimize the flushing symptoms; however, these formulations cost considerably more than ordinary capsules of nicotinic acid. Whatever preparation is used, many people report that the symptoms caused by nicotinic acid begin to lessen after several weeks of continued use. (Note: Nicotinic acid/niacin should not be confused with "niacinamide" or "nicotinamide." The last two preparations will *not* lower blood cholesterol levels.)

Other symptoms—including itching, a burning sensation of the skin, diarrhea, vomiting, and headaches—are also commonly associated with the high doses of nicotinic acid required to lower blood cholesterol levels. On *very rare* occasions, serious liver problems—even leading to death—have occurred when nicotinic acid was taken at doses of 3 grams a day or more. So although nicotinic acid is a vitamin—available without a prescription—you should not use it to lower your cholesterol level without your physician's supervision. The doctor will want to order blood tests to monitor your liver's function if you are using large amounts of nicotinic acid. If you already have liver disease, gout, or a peptic ulcer, he or she may recommend that you not take this vitamin in such high doses.

Bile Acid Sequestrants: Colestipol, Cholestyramine

Colestipol (trade name: Colestid) and cholestyramine (trade name: Questran) fall into a category of drugs called bile acid sequestrants. These drugs work upon compounds called bile acids, which are manufactured by the liver and released into the intestine. Under normal circumstances, these bile acids—which use up a considerable amount of cholesterol in their manufacture—are reabsorbed to some degree into the bloodstream, where they can raise the blood cholesterol level. However, a bile acid sequestering drug will cause them to be eliminated in the stool, thus preventing their return to the bloodstream. This forces the liver to look elsewhere for the substances it needs to manufacture more cholesterol. It ends up using LDL cholesterol, thereby lowering the LDL level in the blood.

With bile acid sequestrants, noticeable declines in blood cholesterol levels occur about a month after the maximum daily dose is reached (usually, these drugs are started at a low dose and gradually increased). Ultimately, drops in LDL cholesterol levels of 15 to 30 percent are common. For example, in the Lipid Research Clinics Coronary Primary Prevention Trial, involving 3,806 middle-aged men, total cholesterol levels fell an average of 13 percent, while LDL concentrations dropped 20 percent (the LDL levels fell while the HDL levels rose slightly, which is a very desirable occurrence). When researchers checked carefully, they discovered that some men had not taken the full dosage. There were even better results in the group of men who did take the *full* dosage of the drug—their LDL levels fell 35 percent. Other studies have shown that bile acid sequestrants can slow the progression of coronary atherosclerosis in some cases.

However, there are still some problems associated with the use of bile acid sequestrants. For instance, they are not easy to take, since they come in powder form (in individual packets or less-expensive bulk cans) and need to be mixed with water or fruit juice. Also, many people who take them complain about their gritty texture and unpleasant taste. Some of these problems may be eliminated now that a chewable bar form of the drug has been introduced. There may be some side effects, including constipation, nausea, bloating, and flatulence; as a result, in patients who have a history of severe constipation (or symptoms of a peptic ulcer, hiatus hernia, or hemorrhoids), many physicians may choose another cholesterol-lowering drug.

Fortunately, however, some of these adverse effects can be minimized; the constipation, for instance, can often be prevented by a high intake of dietary fiber. But when symptoms become very uncomfortable, many people stray from the drug regimen recommended by their doctors, either consuming less than was prescribed or refusing to take the medication at all. Because of the side effects, the unpleasant taste, and the nuisance of having to mix the powder with liquid, patient compliance has been a real problem with bile acid sequestrants. In the Lipid Research Clinics study, published in 1984, only about half of the patients took the full prescribed dose (six packets a day) of cholestyramine; 23 percent used an average of two or less per day.

Also, bear in mind that bile acid sequestrants can interfere with the absorption of a variety of medications (for instance, beta blockers, diuretics, digitoxin, warfarin, and thyroxine). People who must take drugs such as these may be advised to take their dose of bile acid sequestrant several hours before or one hour after taking any other medications.

Lovastatin

In 1987, after several years of research, a new prescription drug called lovastatin (trade name: Mevacor) was released, the first of a new class of drugs that lower cholesterol levels by blocking the production of cholesterol in the liver. Lovastatin does this by interfering with the activity of a liver enzyme (HMG-CoA reductase) that plays an important role in the manufacture of cholesterol. This forces the liver to remove LDL from the bloodstream in order to continue its production of cholesterol. The more LDL that is removed, the greater the decline in total cholesterol levels. This mode of action makes lovastatin an excellent drug for people whose high blood cholesterol counts are caused by overproduction of cholesterol in the liver. It also appears to work well in many people who do not respond to dietary therapy or other drugs.

Lovastatin has fared very well in research studies, consistently decreasing LDL cholesterol levels by 25 to 45 percent. These reductions are greater than those achieved with any other drug. At this level of effectiveness, it is possible to treat people whose blood cholesterol levels are over 300 and reduce them into a truly desirable range. The drug also lowers LDL cholesterol more than HDL, resulting in a better total cholesterol/HDL ratio.

When lovastatin has been used in combination with other drugs, the reductions in LDL cholesterol have been even more dramatic—as much as 45 to 60 percent. These results suggest that some people with severe hereditary problems—who once were almost certain to face premature heart attacks—may now be able to enjoy better health.

Some side effects have been associated with the use of lovastatin, including nausea, fatigue, insomnia, headaches, muscle pains, and skin rashes. However, one recent study found that these symptoms generally were not serious and tended to disappear with time (even though the drug was still being taken). In this study, 2 percent of patients were forced to withdraw from treatment because of side effects.

In some patients (less than 2 percent), lovastatin use must be discontinued because of abnormal changes in blood chemistry tests, which suggest that the liver is unable to deal with the drug (although evidence of liver damage is fortunately lacking). Even so, people who take lovastatin must have regular blood tests to measure their liver function. Also, because of initial reports that lovastatin might promote the development of cataracts, regular eye examinations are advised for people who use the drug; however, follow-up studies have failed to demonstrate any increase in cataract formation among lovastatin users.

Gemfibrozil

Gemfibrozil (trade name: Lopid) falls into a class of drugs called fibric acid derivatives. Although gemfibrozil was originally recommended for lowering triglyceride levels rather than cholesterol, its success at actually reducing the incidence of coronary heart disease in a recent study has created renewed interest in it. In more than 4,000 men with high blood cholesterol, gemfibrozil produced 10 and 11 percent reductions in the average LDL and total cholesterol levels respectively, while causing a significant *increase* (11 percent) in the average HDL level. The net effect was a 34 percent decrease in the incidence of coronary heart disease among the men who took the drug, compared to those who received placebos.

Gemfibrozil is well tolerated by most patients. Some patients report side effects such as abdominal pain, nausea, and diarrhea, and some may develop chemical abnormalities on blood tests related to liver function. People taking gemfibrozil run an increased risk of developing gallstones, and the drug may potentiate the effectiveness of oral anticoagulant medications.

Clofibrate

Clofibrate (trade name: Atromid-S), like gemfibrozil, is a fibric-acid-derivative-drug that has been approved by the FDA for treating high blood triglyceride levels, not cholesterol problems. Its effects are similar to those produced by gemfibrozil, but clofibrate is not commonly prescribed because studies have revealed a disturbingly high incidence of adverse side effects. Nevertheless, some physicians still use this drug to treat high blood cholesterol in selected patients, particularly those who also have seriously elevated blood triglyceride levels.

Probucol

Probucol (trade name: Lorelco) has been used to treat high blood cholesterol, with generally disappointing results. It reduces the LDL cholesterol by about 8 to 15 percent but at the same time causes undesirable drops in the HDL levels—by as much as 25 percent. Because of its modest effect on LDL and its adverse impact on HDL—and also because little is known about its long-term safety—this drug is not often prescribed. Probucol is usually well tolerated; the primary side effects (nausea, flatulence, diarrhea, abdominal pains) occur in less than 5 percent of patients.

MULTIPLE DRUG THERAPY

If a drug you are taking is not reducing your blood cholesterol to acceptable levels, your physician may recommend switching to another drug or using two drugs in combination. As already noted, several studies have measured the effects of such drug combinations, in some cases with dramatic results.

At the University of Southern California, researchers prescribed a combination of colestipol (30 grams a day), niacin (3 to 12 grams a day), and a low-fat, low-cholesterol diet to men who had undergone coronary bypass surgery. In 1987, they reported that after two years of this therapy, average total cholesterol levels had decreased 26 percent (from 246 to 180), LDL levels dropped 43 percent (from 171 to 97), and HDL levels rose 37 percent (from 45 to 61).

In studies that combined a bile acid sequestrant (cholestyramine, colestipol) with nicotinic acid or lovastatin, LDL cholesterol levels were lowered by as much as 45 to 60 percent. When bile acid sequestrants were used in conjunction with probucol or gemfibrozil, blood cholesterol values sometimes fell significantly. Lovastatin has also been used successfully in combination with nicotinic acid to attack LDL cholesterol concentrations.

In addition to increasing drug effectiveness, combining medications may reduce the incidence of adverse side effects, because each drug can be prescribed at a lower dosage than usual. For example, although drugs such as cholestyramine and colestipol can cause constipation at their usual doses, some researchers have reported that this symptom can be eliminated if drugs like probucol or nicotinic acid—which often cause diarrhea—are administered at the same time. Whether or not you need drugs, your doctor can play an important role in helping you keep your blood cholesterol level in a desirable zone. Work with your doctor to develop a personal cholesterol-lowering program that is not only scientifically sound, but also appropriate for your particular needs. That is the best way to *Count Out Cholesterol*.

14

♥   ♥   ♥   ♥

LOOKING TO THE FUTURE

There was a time when we believed that coronary heart disease was an inescapable consequence of aging. Now we know that this is not so. We have learned how to resist the development of coronary heart disease—in many cases, to prevent it entirely. And though some of us are at greater risk than others for this problem, none of us is powerless against it.

To a large degree, we create our own future. It is time to decide what your future shall be with respect to coronary heart disease. The guidelines presented in this book are based on solid scientific evidence, much of which has been cited throughout these pages. Although there are still cynics who claim that cholesterol doesn't count, it does—and there are many dozens of carefully conducted, persuasive studies that prove it.

Though there is no cure for high blood cholesterol, you have within your reach all the tools you need to control it: a rational and effective dietary program for lowering your LDL cholesterol level, several measures for raising your HDL level, and a variety of powerful medications in case these other measures are not sufficient alone.

What is needed now is a lifetime commitment to use these tools. If you are prepared to make that commitment, you *can* control high blood cholesterol and significantly reduce your risk of suffering from coronary heart disease. Make that commitment now, and honor it for the rest of your life.

Take action, also, to reduce any other risk factors that could contribute to the development of coronary heart disease. If you smoke, quit now. If you live a sedentary life, begin a regular program of exercise. Watch your weight and control your blood pressure. With these steps, not only will you reduce your risk of heart disease, you will dramatically improve the quality of your life.

We doctors who care for you also want you to know that we care *about* you. We wish you success as you take control over this very important aspect of your life, and we stand ready to help you anytime you need it.

♥ ♥ ♥ ♥

APPENDIX
General Food Value Charts

Chart 22

The following tables list the SF1, SF2, and cholesterol values for a wide variety of foods. The SF1 and SF2 values are approximately equal to the number of grams of saturated fat and soluble fiber, respectively, in the portion. The cholesterol values are approximately equal to the number of milligrams of cholesterol in each portion. If your portion is larger or smaller, you will have to multiply or divide these values accordingly.

While the values in these charts are estimates, they provide a good reference for selecting foods to meet your daily dietary needs.

The foods are listed alphabetically within each food category. To lower your blood cholesterol level, select foods that are low in saturated fat, low in cholesterol, and high in soluble fiber.

DAIRY PRODUCTS

Food	Portion	SF1	SF2	Chol
Butter, regular	1 pat	2.5	0.0	11
	1 stick, 4 oz.	60.0	0.0	275
Butter, unsalted	1 pat	2.5	0.0	10
	1 stick, 4 oz.	60.0	0.0	250
Cheese				
American, processed	1 oz.	4.5	0.0	20
American, processed cheese food	1 oz.	4.3	0.0	18
American, spread	1 oz.	4.0	0.0	20
Blue	1 oz.	5.2	0.0	21
Brick	1 oz.	5.3	0.0	26
Brie	1 oz.	4.9	0.0	28
Cheddar	1 oz.	5.9	0.0	29
Cottage, creamed	4 oz.	3.0	0.0	20
Cottage, dry curd	4 oz.	.3	0.0	8
Cottage, 2% fat	4 oz.	1.4	0.0	9
Cottage, 1% fat	4 oz.	.5	0.0	5
Cream	4 oz.	24.0	0.0	120
Edam	1 oz.	4.9	0.0	25
Feta	1 oz.	4.2	0.0	25
Fontina	1 oz.	5.4	0.0	32
Goat	1 oz.	7.0	0.0	30
Gouda	1 oz.	4.9	0.0	32
Gruyere	1 oz.	5.3	0.0	31
Monterey Jack	1 oz.	5.3	0.0	25
Mozzarella, whole-milk	1 oz.	3.7	0.0	22
Mozzarella, skim-milk	1 oz.	3.0	0.0	20
Muenster	1 oz.	5.4	0.0	27
Parmesan, grated	1 tbsp.	1.0	0.0	4
Provolone	1 oz.	4.8	0.0	19
Ricotta, whole-milk	½ cup	9.5	0.0	60
Ricotta, part-skim	½ cup	5.5	0.0	30
Romano	1 oz.	4.8	0.0	29
Roquefort	1 oz.	5.4	0.0	25
Swiss	1 oz.	5.0	0.0	26

Food	Portion	SF1	SF2	Chol
Coffee whitener, powdered	1 tsp.	.5	0.0	0
Cream, half and half	1 tbsp.	1.0	0.0	10
Cream, light, table	1 tbsp.	1.8	0.0	10
Cream, light, whipping	1 tbsp.	2.9	0.0	17
Cream, heavy, whipping	1 tbsp.	3.5	0.0	21
Cream, whip, pressurized	1 tbsp.	.4	0.0	2
Milk				
Low-fat, 2%	1 cup	3.0	0.0	20
Skim	1 cup	.3	0.0	4
Whole, 3.3% fat	1 cup	5.0	0.0	30
Buttermilk, cultured	1 cup	1.5	0.0	10
Chocolate, whole	1 cup	5.5	.1	30
Chocolate, 2% low-fat	1 cup	3.1	.1	17
Condensed, sweet	1 oz.	2.1	0.0	13
Dry, whole	1 cup	21.4	0.0	124
Dry, non-fat, regular	1 cup	.6	0.0	24
Dry, non-fat, instant	1 cup	.3	0.0	12
Evaporated, whole	½ cup	5.8	0.0	37
Evaporated, skim	½ cup	.2	0.0	5
Goat, whole	1 cup	6.5	0.0	28
Imitation, with vegetable oil	1 cup	1.9	0.0	0
Cocoa, homemade	1 cup	5.5	.1	30
Malted milk powder, natural flavor	.75 oz. (2 to 3 tsp.)	.9	0.0	4
Malted milk powder, chocolate	.75 oz. (2 to 3 tsp.)	.5	.4	1
Milk shake, chocolate (fastfood)	10 oz.	6.5	0.2	40
Milk shake, strawberry (fastfood)	10 oz.	4.9	0.0	31
Milk shake, vanilla (fastfood)	10 oz.	5.3	0.0	31
Sour cream	1 tbsp.	1.6	0.0	5
Sour cream, imitation	1 oz.	5.0	0.0	0
Yogurt, plain	4 oz.	2.5	0.0	15
Yogurt, low-fat	4 oz.	1.1	0.0	7
Yogurt, skim	4 oz.	.1	0.0	2
Yogurt, fruit, low-fat	4 oz.	.8	0.0	5

Food	Portion	SF1	SF2	Chol
Egg, chicken, whole, raw	1 large egg	1.5	0.0	270
Egg, chicken, white, raw	1 large egg white	0.0	0.0	0
Egg, chicken, yolk, raw	1 large egg yolk	1.6	0.0	213
Egg, duck, whole	1 egg	2.6	0.0	619
Egg, goose, whole	1 egg	5.2	0.0	1227
Egg substitute, frozen	¼ cup	1.2	0.0	1
Egg substitute, powder	0.7 oz.	.7	0.0	113
Eggnog	1 cup	11.5	0.0	149

CEREALS

Food	Portion	SF1	SF2	Chol
All-bran, ready-to-eat	1 oz.	0.0	3.0	0
Alpha-bits	1 oz.	0.0	.4	0
Apple Jacks	1 oz.	0.0	.2	0
Bran Buds	1 oz.	0.0	3.2	0
Bran Chex	1 oz.	0.0	1.4	0
C.W. Post, plain	1 oz.	3.3	.6	0
C.W. Post, with raisins	1 oz.	3.0	1.1	0
Cap'n Crunch	1 oz.	1.7	.2	0
Cap'n Crunch, crunchberrys	1 oz.	1.6	.2	0
Cap'n Crunch, peanut butter	1 oz.	1.5	.1	0
Cheerios	1 oz.	.3	.6	0
Cocoa Krispies	1 oz.	0.0	.1	0
Cocoa Pebbles	1 oz.	0.0	.1	0
Cookiecrisp	1 oz.	0.0	.1	0
Corn Bran	1 oz.	0.0	1.6	0
Corn Chex	1 oz.	0.0	.2	0
Corn Flakes, Kellogg's	1 oz.	0.0	0.2	0
Corn Flakes, Ralston-Purina	1 oz.	0.0	0.2	0
Cracklin' Oat Bran	1 oz.	0.0	1.4	0
Cream of Rice, cooked	1 cup	0.0	.1	0
Cream of Wheat, instant, cooked	1 cup	0.0	.9	0
Cream of Wheat, regular, cooked	1 cup	0.0	.5	0
Cream of Wheat, quick, cooked	1 cup	0.0	.4	0

Food	Portion	SF1	SF2	Chol
Crispy Rice	1 oz.	0.0	.1	0
Crispy Wheats'n Raisins	1 oz.	0.0	.6	0
Farina, cooked	1 cup	0.0	1.0	0
Fortified Oat Flakes	1 oz.	0.0	.3	0
40% Bran Flakes, Kellogg's	1 oz.	0.2	1.0	0
40% Bran Flakes, Post	1 oz.	0.2	1.0	0
Froot Loops	1 oz.	0.0	.2	0
Frosted Mini-Wheats	1 oz.	0.0	.6	0
Frosted Rice Krinkles	1 oz.	0.0	.1	0
Frosted Rice Krispies	1 oz.	0.0	.1	0
Fruity Pebbles	1 oz.	0.0	.1	0
Golden Grahams	1 oz.	.7	.3	0
Graham Crackos	1 oz.	0.0	.5	0
Grape-Nuts	1 oz.	0.0	.9	0
Grape-Nuts Flakes	1 oz.	0.0	.8	0
Grits, yellow, cooked	1 cup	.1	.1	0
Grits, white, cooked	1 cup	.1	.1	0
Heartland Natural, plain	1 oz.	0.0	.5	0
Heartland Natural, with coconut	1 oz.	0.0	.6	0
Heartland Natural, with raisins	1 oz.	0.0	.5	0
Honey+Nut Corn Flakes	1 oz.	0.0	.1	0
Honeybran Cereal	1 oz.	0.0	.9	0
Honey Nut Cheerios	1 oz.	.1	.4	0
Honeycomb	1 oz.	0.0	.2	0
King Vitaman	1 oz.	1.0	.1	0
Kix	1 oz.	.2	.2	0
Life, plain/cinnamon	1 oz.	0.0	.5	0
Lucky Charms	1 oz.	.2	.4	0
Maltex, cooked	1 cup	0.0	.9	0
Malt-O-Meal, cooked	1 cup	0.0	.3	0
Maypo, cooked	1 cup	0.0	1.7	0
Most	1 oz.	0.0	1.2	0
Nature Valley Granola	1 oz.	.8	.5	0
Nutri-Grain, barley	1 oz.	0.0	.5	0
Nutri-Grain, corn	1 oz.	0.0	.5	0
Nutri-Grain, rye	1 oz.	0.0	.5	0
Nutri-Grain, wheat	1 oz.	0.0	.5	0
Oats, rolled, cooked	1 cup	.4	2.0	0

COUNT OUT CHOLESTEROL

Food	Portion	SF1	SF2	Chol
100% Bran	1 oz.	.2	5.0	0
100% Natural, plain	1 oz.	4.1	.7	0
100% Natural, with apple+cinnamon	1 oz.	4.2	.6	0
100% Natural, with raisins+dates	1 oz.	3.5	.6	0
Product 19	1 oz.	0.0	.3	0
Quisp	1 oz.	1.4	.2	0
Raisin Bran, Kellogg's	1 oz.	0.1	1.0	0
Raisin Bran, Post	1 oz.	0.1	1.0	0
Raisin Bran, Ralston-Purina	1 oz.	0.1	1.1	0
Raisins, rice+rye	1 oz.	0.0	.5	0
Ralston, cooked	1 cup	0.0	1.8	0
Roman Meal, cooked	1 cup	0.0	0.0	0
Rice Chex	1 oz.	0.0	.2	0
Rice Krispies	1 oz.	0.0	.1	0
Rice, puffed	1 oz.	0.0	.2	0
Special K	1 oz.	0.0	.2	0
Sugar Corn Pops	1 oz.	0.0	.1	0
Sugar Frosted Flakes, Kellogg's	1 oz.	0.0	.2	0
Sugar Frosted Flakes, Ralston-Purina	1 oz.	0.0	.2	0
Sugar Smacks	1 oz.	0.0	.1	0
Sugar Sparkled Flakes	1 oz.	0.0	.1	0
Super Sugar Crisp	1 oz.	0.0	.1	0
Tasteeos	1 oz.	0.0	.9	0
Team	1 oz.	0.0	.1	0
Toasties	1 oz.	0.0	.3	0
Total	1 oz.	.1	1.1	0
Trix	1 oz.	0.0	.1	0
Waffelos	1 oz.	0.0	0.0	0
Wheat 'n Raisin Chex	1 oz.	0.0	.6	0
Wheat Chex	1 oz.	0.0	.8	0
Wheatena, cooked	1 cup	0.0	2.0	0
Wheat Germ, toasted	1 oz.	.5	1.1	0
Wheat Germ, toasted, with sugar	1 oz.	.4	.4	0
Wheaties	1 oz.	.1	.7	0
Wheat, puffed	1 cup	0.0	.2	0

Food	Portion	SF1	SF2	Chol
Wheat, shredded, large biscuit	1 rectangular biscuit	0.0	.7	0
Wheat, shredded, small biscuit	1 cup	0.2	.5	0

BREADS, CRACKERS, AND WAFFLES

Food	Portion	SF1	SF2	Chol
Bagels				
Cinnamon-raisin	3.5"	.2	0.0	0
Cinnamon-raisin, toasted	3.5"	.2	0.0	0
Egg	3.5"	.3	0.0	17
Egg, toasted	3.5"	.3	0.0	17
Oatbran	3.5"	.1	0.0	0
Oatbran, toasted	3.5"	.1	0.0	0
Plain	3.5"	.3	.5	0
Plain, toasted	3.5"	.3	0.0	0
Biscuit, plain, dry mix, prepared	1 biscuit	1.6	.3	2
Biscuit, mixed-grain, refrigerator dough, baked	1 biscuit	.7	0.0	0
Breads				
Banana, with margarine	1 slice	1.3	0.0	26
Banana, with vegetable shortening	1 slice	1.8	0.0	26
Cornbread, dry mix, prepared	1 piece	1.6	.4	37
Cracked-wheat	1 slice	.2	.4	0
Cracked-wheat, toasted	1 slice	.2	0.0	0
Egg	1 slice	.6	0.0	20
Egg, toasted	1 slice	.6	0.0	21
Indian (Navajo), fried	5" diameter	1.7	0.0	0
Irish Soda	1 slice	.7	0.0	11
Italian	1 slice	.3	.3	0
Italian, toasted	1 slice	.3	0.0	0
Mixed-grain	1 slice	.2	.6	0
Mixed-grain, toasted	1 slice	.2	0.0	0
Oat Bran	1 slice	.2	.5	0

Food	Portion	SF1	SF2	Chol
Oat Bran, toasted	1 slice	.2	0.0	0
Oat Bran, reduced-calorie	1 slice	.1	0.0	0
Oatmeal	1 slice	.2	.3	0
Oatmeal, toasted	1 slice	.2	0.0	0
Pita, white	1 pita	.1	.5	0
Pita, whole-wheat	1 pita	.3	1.4	0
Protein	1 slice	.1	0.0	0
Pumpernickel	1 slice	.1	.6	0
Pumpernickel, toasted	1 slice	.1	0.0	0
Pumpkin	1 slice	1.2	0.0	26
Raisin	1 slice	.3	.3	0
Raisin, toasted	1 slice	.3	0.0	0
Rye	1 slice	.2	.6	0
Rye, toasted	1 slice	.2	0.0	0
Rye, reduced-calorie	1 slice	.1	0.0	0
Wheat	1 slice	.2	.3	0
Wheat, toasted	1 slice	.2	0.0	0
Wheat, reduced-calorie	1 slice	.1	.8	0
Wheat bran	1 slice	.3	.9	0
Wheat bran, toasted	1 slice	.3	0.0	0
White	1 slice	.3	.3	0
White, toasted	1 slice	.3	0.0	0
White, reduced-calorie	1 slice	.1	.6	0
Whole wheat	1 slice	.4	0.3	0
Whole wheat, toasted	1 slice	.3	.6	0
Breadcrumbs, dry, plain	1 cup	1.4	1.4	0
Breadsticks, plain	1 stick	.1	0.0	0
Bread stuffing, dry mix, prepared	½ cup	1.7	.9	0
Bread stuffing, corn, dry mix, prepared	½ cup	1.8	0.0	0
Crackers				
Cheese	1" square cracker	.1	0.0	0
Cheese+peanut butter	1 sandwich cracker	.4	0.0	0
Cheese, sandwich	1 sandwich cracker	.4	0.0	0
Crisp bread, rye	1 wafer	0.0	.5	0
Matzo, plain	1 matzo (1 oz.)	.1	.3	0
Matzo, egg	1 matzo (1 oz.)	.2	0.0	25

Food	Portion	SF1	SF2	Chol
Matzo, whole wheat	1 matzo (1 oz.)	.1	1.0	0
Melba toast, plain	1 toast	.1	.1	0
Melba toast, rye	1 toast	.1	.1	0
Melba toast, wheat	1 toast	.1	.1	0
Milk	1 cracker	.4	0.0	2
Peanut butter	1 sandwich cracker	.4	0.0	0
Rye+cheese	1 sandwich cracker	.4	0.0	1
Rye wafers, plain	1 triple cracker	0.0	0.0	0
Rye wafers, sandwich	1 triple cracker	.3	0.0	0
Saltines	1 saltine	.1	0.0	2
Wheat, regular	1 thin square cracker	.1	0.0	0
Wheat+cheese	1 sandwich cracker	.5	0.0	0
Wheat+peanut butter	1 sandwich cracker	.4	0.0	0
Whole wheat	1 square cracker	.2	.1	0
Cracker meal	1 cup	.3	0.0	0
Croissants, apple	1 medium	2.5	.4	29
Croissants, butter	1 medium	6.7	.5	43
Croissants, cheese	1 medium	5.5	.6	36
Croutons, plain	1 cup	.5	.5	0
Croutons, seasoned	1 cup	2.0	.6	1
English muffin, plain, toasted	1 muffin	.3	0.5	0
English muffin, mixed-grain	1 muffin	.2	0.0	0
English muffin, raisin-cinnamon	1 muffin	.2	0.0	0
English muffin, whole wheat	1 muffin	.2	1.2	0
French Toast, frozen, ready-to-heat	1 piece	1.1	.5	48
French Toast, 2% milk	1 piece	1.8	0.0	75
Muffin, plain, 2% milk	1 muffin	1.2	.5	22
Muffin, blueberry	1 muffin	.7	.6	17
Muffin, corn	1 muffin	1.5	.5	20
Muffin, oat bran	1 muffin	.5	1.3	0
Muffin, wheat bran, dry mix, prepared	1 muffin	1.5	0.5	20
Pancake, plain, dry mix, prepared	4" pancake	.2	.1	5
Pancake, plain, frozen, ready-to-heat	4" pancake	.3	0.0	3

Food	Portion	SF1	SF2	Chol
Pancake, buckwheat, dry mix, prepared	4" pancake	.6	.2	20
Pancake, buttermilk	4" pancake	.7	0.0	22
Pancake, whole wheat, dry mix, prepared	4" pancake	.8	0.0	27
Roll, dinner, egg	1 roll	.6	.4	18
Roll, dinner, oat bran	1 roll	.2	.4	0
Roll, dinner, rye	1 roll	.2	0.0	0
Roll, dinner, wheat	1 roll	.4	0.0	0
Roll, dinner, whole wheat	1 roll	.2	0.0	0
Roll, french	1 roll	.4	0.0	0
Roll, hamburger/hot dog	1 roll	.5	0.5	0
Roll, hamburger/hot dog, mixed-grain	1 roll	.5	.5	0
Roll, hard	1 roll	.3	0.0	0
Taco shells, baked	1 medium	.4	.3	0
Tortillas, ready-to-bake, fried, corn	1 medium	.1	1.0	0
Tortillas, ready-to-bake, fried, flour	1 medium	.4	.3	0
Waffles, plain, dry mix, complete	1 waffle	1.7	.3	38
Waffles, plain, frozen, ready-to-heat	1 waffle	.5	.3	8
Waffles, home-made	1 waffle	4.0	.5	100
Waffles, buttermilk	1 waffle	1.9	0.0	50
Wonton wrappers	1 wonton wrapper	0.0	0.0	1

GRAINS AND PASTA

Food	Portion	SF1	SF2	Chol
Amaranth	1 cup	3.2	8.9	0
Arrowroot	1 cup	0.0	1.3	0
Barley	1 cup	.9	9.5	0
Buckwheat	1 cup	1.3	5.1	0
Buckwheat flour, whole	1 cup	.8	3.6	0
Bulgur, cooked	1 cup	.5	.2	0
Corn bran, crude	1 cup	.1	19.6	0
Corn flour, whole, yellow	1 cup	.6	4.7	0

Food	Portion	SF1	SF2	Chol
Corn flour, whole, white	1 cup	.6	3.4	0
Corn flour, masa, enriched	1 cup	.6	3.3	0
Cornmeal, whole, yellow	1 cup	.6	2.7	0
Cornmeal, degermed, enriched, yellow	1 cup	.2	4.0	0
Cornstarch	1 cup	0.0	.3	0
Couscous, cooked	1 cup	.1	.8	0
Hominy, canned, white	1 cup	.2	1.2	0
Millet	1 cup	1.4	5.1	0
Oat bran, raw	1 cup	1.2	4.4	0
Oat bran, cooked	1 cup	.4	0.0	0
Oats	1 cup	1.9	0.0	0
Quinoa	1 cup	1.0	3.0	0
Rice bran, crude	1 cup	3.5	5.2	0
Rice, brown, long, cooked	1 cup	.4	1.1	0
Rice, brown, medium, cooked	1 cup	.3	.4	0
Rice, white, long, cooked	1 cup	.1	.2	0
Rice, white, medium, cooked	1 cup	.1	.2	0
Rice, white, short, cooked	1 cup	.1	0.0	0
Rice, white, instant, enriched, cooked	1 cup	.1	.2	0
Rice, wild, cooked	1 cup	.1	.9	0
Rice flour, brown	1 cup	.9	2.2	0
Rice flour, white	1 cup	.6	1.1	0
Rye	1 cup	.5	7.4	0
Rye flour, dark	1 cup	.4	8.7	0
Rye flour, light	1 cup	.1	4.5	0
Rye flour, medium	1 cup	.2	4.5	0
Semolina, enriched	1 cup	.3	2.0	0
Sorghum	1 cup	.9	0.0	0
Tapioca, pearl, dry	1 cup	0.0	.4	0
Triticale	1 cup	.7	0.0	0
Triticale flour	1 cup	.4	5.7	0
Wheat, hard, red	1 cup	.5	7.3	0
Wheat, soft, red	1 cup	.5	0.0	0
Wheat, hard, white	1 cup	.5	0.0	0
Wheat, soft, white	1 cup	.6	0.0	0
Wheat, durum	1 cup	.9	0.0	0
Wheat bran, crude	1 cup	.4	7.8	0

Food	Portion	SF1	SF2	Chol
Wheat germ, crude	1 cup	1.7	4.0	0
Wheat flour, whole	1 cup	.4	4.4	0
Wheat, sprouted	1 cup	.2	.4	0
White flour, enriched, all purpose, bleached	1 cup	.3	2.0	0
White flour, bread	1 cup	.3	1.0	0
White flour, cake, enriched	1 cup	.1	.6	0
White flour, tortilla, mix	1 cup	4.6	0.0	0
Macaroni, enriched, cooked	1 cup	.1	.3	0
Macaroni, protein-fortified, cooked	1 cup	0.0	0.0	0
Macaroni, vegetable, enriched, cooked	1 cup	0.0	1.7	0
Macaroni, whole wheat, cooked	1 cup	.1	1.8	0
Noodle, egg, enriched, cooked	1 cup	.5	.5	50
Noodle, egg, spinach, cooked	1 cup	.6	1.1	53
Noodle, Chow Mein	1 cup	2.0	.5	0
Noodle, Japanese, soba, cooked	1 cup	0.0	0.0	0
Noodle, Japanese, somen, cooked	1 cup	0.0	0.0	0
Pasta, corn, cooked	1 cup	.1	2.0	0
Pasta, fresh, cooked	1 cup	.4	0.0	66
Pasta, fresh, spinach, cooked	1 cup	.4	0.0	66
Pasta with egg, cooked	1 cup	.8	0.0	82
Pasta, no egg, cooked	1 cup	.2	0.0	0
Spaghetti, enriched, cooked	1 cup	.1	.5	0
Spaghetti, spinach, cooked	1 cup	.1	0.0	0
Spaghetti, whole wheat, cooked	1 cup	.1	1.9	0

NUTS AND SEEDS

Food	Portion	SF1	SF2	Chol
Almond butter	1 tbsp.	.9	.2	0
Almond butter, honey+cinnamon	1 tbsp.	.8	0.0	0

Food	Portion	SF1	SF2	Chol
Almonds, dried	1 oz.	1.4	.9	0
Almonds, dried, blanched	1 oz.	1.4	.6	0
Almonds, dry roasted	1 oz.	1.4	1.2	0
Almonds, honey roasted	1 oz.	1.3	0.0	0
Almonds, oil roasted	1 oz.	1.6	1.0	0
Almonds, oil roasted, blanched	1 oz.	1.5	1.0	0
Almonds, toasted	1 oz.	1.4	1.0	0
Almond paste	1 oz.	.7	1.3	0
Beechnuts, dried	1 oz.	1.6	0.0	0
Brazil nuts, dried	1 oz.	4.5	.4	0
Breadfruit seed, roasted	1 oz.	.2	0.0	0
Butternuts, dried	1 oz.	.4	.4	0
Cashew butter	1 oz.	2.8	.2	0
Cashews, dry roasted	1 oz.	2.5	.3	0
Cashews, oil roasted	1 oz.	2.7	.3	0
Chestnuts, Chinese, raw	1 oz.	0.0	0.0	0
Chestnuts, Chinese, boiled	1 oz.	0.0	0.0	0
Chestnuts, Chinese, dried	1 oz.	.1	0.0	0
Chestnuts, Chinese, roasted	1 oz.	0.0	0.0	0
Chestnuts, European, boiled	1 oz.	.1	0.0	0
Chestnuts, European, dry, peeled	1 oz.	.2	0.0	0
Chestnuts, European, raw, peeled	1 oz.	.1	0.0	0
Chestnuts, European, roasted	1 oz.	.1	1.1	0
Chia seeds, dried	1 oz.	3.0	0.0	0
Filberts, dried	1 oz.	1.3	.5	0
Filberts, dried, blanched	1 oz.	1.4	0.0	0
Filberts, dry roasted	1 oz.	1.4	0.0	0
Filberts, oil roasted	1 oz.	1.3	.5	0
Ginkgo nuts, canned	1 oz.	.1	.8	0
Ginkgo nuts, dried	1 oz.	.1	0.0	0
Ginkgo nuts, raw	1 oz.	.1	0.0	0
Hickory nuts, dried	1 oz.	2.0	.5	0
Lotus seeds, dried	1 oz.	.1	0.0	0
Lotus seeds, raw	1 oz.	0.0	0.0	0

COUNT OUT CHOLESTEROL

Food	Portion	SF1	SF2	Chol
Macadamia nuts, dried	1 oz.	3.0	.8	0
Macadamia nuts, oil roasted	1 oz.	3.3	0.0	0
Mixed nuts/peanut, dry roasted	1 oz.	2.0	.8	0
Mixed nuts/peanut, oil roasted	1 oz.	2.5	.8	0
Mixed nuts, oil roasted	1 oz.	2.6	0.0	0
Peanut butter, with salt	1 tbsp.	1.5	.1	0
Peanuts, oil roasted, with salt	1 oz.	2.0	0.0	0
Pecans, dried	1 oz.	1.5	.3	0
Pecans, dry roasted	1 oz.	1.5	0.0	0
Pecans, oil roasted	1 oz.	1.6	0.0	0
Pilinuts, dried	1 oz.	8.9	0.0	0
Pine pignolias, dried	1 oz.	2.2	.4	0
Pine nut, pinyon, dried	1 oz.	2.7	.9	0
Pistachio nuts, dried	1 oz.	1.7	.9	0
Pistachio nuts, dry roasted	1 oz.	1.9	.9	0
Pumpkin seeds, dried	1 oz.	2.5	1.2	0
Pumpkin seeds, roasted	1 oz.	2.3	0.0	0
Safflower seed, dried	1 oz.	1.0	0.0	0
Sesame butter paste	1 oz.	2.0	.5	0
Sesame seed, whole, dried	1 oz.	1.3	.6	0
Sesame seed, whole, roasted	1 oz.	1.9	1.2	0
Soybean kernel, roasted	1 oz.	.9	.3	0
Sunflower kernel, dry roasted, with salt	1 oz.	1.5	.6	0
Sunflower kernel, oil roasted, with salt	1 oz.	1.7	.6	0
Sunflower kernel, toasted, with salt	1 oz.	1.7	0.0	0
Tahini, raw kernels	1 oz.	1.9	.8	0
Tahini, roasted kernels	1 oz.	2.1	.8	0
Walnuts, black, dried	1 oz.	1.0	.4	0
Walnuts, English, dried	1 oz.	1.5	.2	0
Wheatnuts, formulated	1 oz.	2.5	.4	0

VEGETABLES

Food	Portion	SF1	SF2	Chol
Alfalfa, sprouted, raw	½ cup	0.0	.1	0
Amaranth, raw	½ cup	0.0	0.0	0
Arrowhead, raw	1 medium corn	0.0	0.0	0
Artichoke, raw	1 medium	0.0	2.1	0
Artichoke, boiled	1 medium	0.0	1.9	0
Asparagus, raw	½ cup	0.0	.6	0
Asparagus, boiled	½ cup	0.0	.5	0
Asparagus, frozen, boiled	4 spears	0.0	.5	0
Balsam-pear leaf, boiled	½ cup	0.0	.2	0
Balsam-pear pod, boiled	½ cup	0.0	.4	0
Bamboo shoots, raw	½ cup	.1	.5	0
Bamboo shoots, boiled	½ cup	.1	0.0	0
Bean sprouts, kidney, raw	½ cup	.1	0.0	0
Bean sprouts, kidney, boiled	½ cup	.1	0.0	0
Bean, lima, raw	½ cup	.2	1.1	0
Bean, lima, boiled	½ cup	.1	1.4	0
Bean, lima, baby, frozen, boiled	½ cup	.1	0.0	0
Bean, lima, ford, frozen, boiled	½ cup	.1	1.8	0
Bean sprout, mung, raw	½ cup	0.0	.3	0
Bean sprout, mung, boiled	½ cup	0.0	.1	0
Bean, pinto, frozen, boiled	½ cup	.1	0.0	0
Bean, snap, green, raw	½ cup	0.0	.5	0
Bean, snap, green, boiled	½ cup	0.0	.5	0
Bean, snap, green, frozen, boiled	½ cup	0.0	.6	0
Bean, snap, yellow, boiled	½ cup	0.0	.2	0
Bean, snap, yellow, canned, solid+liquid	½ cup	0.0	.3	0
Bean, snap, yellow, frozen, boiled	½ cup	0.0	0.0	0
Beets, raw	½ cup	0.0	1.2	0
Beets, cooked, boiled, drained	½ cup	0.0	1.0	0
Beet greens, raw	½ cup	0.0	.2	0
Beet greens, boiled	½ cup	0.0	.6	0
Broadbeans, raw	½ cup	.1	.7	0

Food	Portion	SF1	SF2	Chol
Broadbeans, boiled	½ cup	.1	0.0	0
Broccoli, raw	½ cup	.1	1.0	0
Broccoli, cooked, boiled	½ cup	.1	1.0	0
Broccoli, frozen, chopped, boiled	½ cup	.1	.8	0
Brussels sprouts, raw	½ cup	.1	1.5	0
Brussel sprouts, boiled	½ cup	.1	1.5	0
Brussel sprouts, frozen, boiled	½ cup	.1	1.0	0
Cabbage, raw	½ cup	0.0	.4	0
Cabbage, cooked, boiled, drained	½ cup	0.0	.5	0
Cabbage, red, raw	½ cup	0.0	.4	0
Cabbage, red, boiled	½ cup	0.0	.5	0
Cabbage, pak-choi, raw	½ cup	0.0	.1	0
Cabbage, pak-choi, boiled	½ cup	0.0	.4	0
Carrots, raw	½ cup	0.0	1.0	0
Carrots, boiled	½ cup	0.0	1.0	0
Carrots, frozen, boiled	½ cup	0.0	1.0	0
Carrot juice, canned	½ cup	0.0	.3	0
Cauliflower, raw	½ cup	0.0	.4	0
Cauliflower, boiled, drained	½ cup	0.0	.5	0
Cauliflower, frozen, boiled	½ cup	0.0	.6	0
Celeriac, raw	½ cup	0.0	.4	0
Celeriac, boiled	½ cup	0.0	0.0	0
Celery, raw	½ cup	0.0	.4	0
Celery, boiled	½ cup	0.0	.5	0
Chard, swiss, raw	½ cup	0.0	.1	0
Chard, swiss, boiled	½ cup	0.0	.6	0
Chicory, witloof, raw	½ cup	0.0	.4	0
Chicory greens, raw	½ cup	.1	1.1	0
Chicory roots, raw	½ cup	0.0	0.0	0
Chives, raw	1 tbsp.	0.0	0.0	0
Collards, raw	½ cup	0.0	.2	0
Collards, boiled	½ cup	0.0	.4	0
Collards, frozen, boiled	½ cup	0.0	0.0	0
Corn, sweet, yellow, boiled	½ cup	.2	.7	0
Corn, yellow, canned, drained	½ cup	.1	.5	0

Food	Portion	SF1	SF2	Chol
Corn, yellow, canned, cream style	½ cup	.1	.5	0
Corn, yellow, frozen, boiled	½ cup	0.0	.6	0
Corn, red+green pepper, canned	½ cup	.1	0.0	0
Corn, white, boiled	½ cup	0.0	1.5	0
Corn, white, canned, drained	½ cup	.1	.3	0
Corn, white, canned, cream style	½ cup	.1	.5	0
Cornsalad, raw	½ cup	0.0	0.0	0
Cowpeas, raw	½ cup	.1	1.1	0
Cowpeas, boiled	½ cup	.1	1.2	0
Cowpeas, frozen, boiled	½ cup	.1	0.0	0
Cucumber, raw	½ cup	0.0	.2	0
Dandelion greens, raw	½ cup	0.0	.3	0
Dandelion greens, boiled	½ cup	0.0	.5	0
Eggplant, raw	½ cup	0.0	.9	0
Eggplant, boiled	½ cup	0.0	1.0	0
Endive, raw	½ cup	0.0	.2	0
Fennel, bulb, raw	½ cup	0.0	0.0	0
Garlic, raw	1 clove	0.0	0.0	0
Ginger root, raw	½ cup	0.0	.2	0
Horseradish-leaf, raw	½ cup	0.0	.1	0
Horseradish-leaf, cooked	½ cup	0.0	.1	0
Kale, raw	½ cup	0.0	.2	0
Kale, boiled	½ cup	0.0	.4	0
Kale, frozen, boiled	½ cup	0.0	0.0	0
Kohlrabi, raw	½ cup	0.0	.8	0
Kohlrabi, boiled	½ cup	0.0	.3	0
Leeks, raw	½ cup	0.0	.2	0
Leeks, boiled	½ cup	0.0	0.0	0
Lentils, sprouted, raw	½ cup	0.0	0.0	0
Lettuce, butterhead, raw	1 head, 5" diameter	0.0	.5	0
Lettuce, iceberg, raw	1 head, 6" diameter	.1	2.3	0
Lettuce, looseleaf, raw	½ cup	0.0	.2	0
Lettuce, romaine, raw	½ cup	0.0	.2	0
Lotus root, raw	10 slices, 2½" diameter	0.0	1.2	0

Food	Portion	SF1	SF2	Chol
Lotus root, boiled	10 slices, 2½" diameter	0.0	.8	0
Mushrooms, raw	½ cup	0.0	.3	0
Mushrooms, boiled	½ cup	0.0	.5	0
Mushrooms, canned, drained	½ cup	0.0	.6	0
Mushrooms, shitake, cooked	4 mushrooms	0.0	.5	0
Mushrooms, shitake, dried	4 mushrooms	0.0	.5	0
Mustard greens, raw	½ cup	0.0	.2	0
Mustard greens, boiled	½ cup	0.0	.4	0
Mustard greens, frozen, boiled	½ cup	0.0	0.0	0
Okra, raw	½ cup	0.0	.4	0
Okra, boiled	½ cup	0.0	.6	0
Okra, frozen, boiled	½ cup	.1	.8	0
Onions, raw	½ cup	0.1	1.0	0
Onions, boiled	½ cup	0.0	1.0	0
Onions, canned, solid+liquid	½ cup	0.0	1.0	0
Parsley, raw	½ cup	0.0	.3	0
Parsnips, raw	½ cup	0.0	1.0	0
Parsnips, boiled	½ cup	0.0	.9	0
Peas, edible pod, raw	½ cup	0.0	.6	0
Peas, edible pod, boiled	½ cup	0.0	.7	0
Peas, edible pod, frozen, boiled	½ cup	.1	0.0	0
Peas, green, raw	½ cup	.1	2.0	0
Peas, green, boiled	½ cup	.1	2.0	0
Peas, green, canned, solid+liquid	½ cup	.1	1.0	0
Peas, green, canned, drained	½ cup	.1	.9	0
Peas, green, frozen, boiled	½ cup	0.0	1.3	0
Peas, sprouted, raw	½ cup	.1	0.0	0
Peas, sprouted, boiled	½ cup	.1	0.0	0
Peas+carrots, canned, solid+liquid	½ cup	.1	1.3	0
Peas+carrots, frozen, boiled	½ cup	.1	.9	0

Food	Portion	SF1	SF2	Chol
Peas+onions, canned, solid+liquid	½ cup	0.0	0.0	0
Peas+onions, frozen, boiled	½ cup	0.0	.8	0
Peppers, hot chili, raw	½ cup	0.0	.3	0
Peppers, sweet, raw	½ cup	0.0	.3	0
Peppers, sweet, boiled	½ cup	0.0	.2	0
Poi	½ cup	0.0	.1	0
Potatoes, peeled, raw	½ cup	0.0	.4	0
Potatoes, with skin, baked	1 medium	0.1	2.0	0
Potatoes, boiled, unpeeled	½ cup	0.0	.4	0
Potatoes, boiled, peeled	½ cup	0.0	.4	0
Potatoes, hash brown	½ cup	4.2	.5	0
Potatoes, mashed, with milk+butter	½ cup	3.2	0.0	15
Potatoes, mashed, with milk+margarine	½ cup	1.1	.6	2
Potatoes, scalloped, home	½ cup	2.8	.7	15
Potatoes, au gratin, home	½ cup	5.8	.7	28
Potato flakes, no milk, prepared	½ cup	3.6	.7	15
Potato puffs, frozen, prepared	½ cup	3.2	.6	0
Potatoes, frozen, fried, vegetable oil	10 strips	2.5	.2	0
Pumpkin, raw	½ cup	0.0	.3	0
Pumpkin, boiled	½ cup	0.0	0.0	0
Pumpkin, canned	½ cup	.2	1.0	0
Raddicchio, raw	½ cup	0.0	0.0	0
Radishes, raw	½ cup	0.0	.3	0
Radishes, oriental, raw	½ cup	0.0	.2	0
Radishes, oriental, boiled	½ cup	.1	.4	0
Rutabaga, raw	½ cup	0.0	.5	0
Rutabaga, boiled	½ cup	0.0	.5	0
Sauerkraut, canned, solid+liquid	½ cup	0.1	1.0	0
Seaweed, agar, dried	½ cup	.1	2.3	0
Seaweed, spirulina, raw	½ cup	.1	0.0	0
Seaweed, spirulina, drained	½ cup	2.7	1.1	0
Seaweed, wakame, raw	½ cup	.1	.2	0

Food	Portion	SF1	SF2	Chol
Shallots, raw	1 tbsp.	0.0	0.0	
Soybeans, green, raw	½ cup	1.0	1.6	0
Soybeans, green, boiled	½ cup	.7	1.1	0
Soybeans, sprouts, raw	½ cup	.3	0.0	0
Soybeans, sprouts, steamed	½ cup	.3	.1	0
Soybeans, sprouts, stir-fry	½ cup	1.0	0.0	0
Spinach, raw	½ cup	0.0	.2	0
Spinach, boiled	½ cup	0.1	.5	0
Spinach, frozen, boiled	½ cup	0.0	.9	0
Squash, acorn, baked	½ cup	0.3	0.4	0
Squash, butternut, baked	½ cup	0.0	0.0	0
Squash, crookneck, boiled	½ cup	.1	.3	0
Squash, hubbard, baked	½ cup	.1	0.0	0
Squash, spaghetti, boiled	½ cup	0.0	.3	0
Squash, zucchini, boiled	½ cup	0.1	1.5	0
Squash, zucchini, frozen, boiled	½ cup	0.0	0.0	0
Succotash, boiled	½ cup	.1	0.0	0
Succotash, frozen, boiled	½ cup	.1	1.4	0
Sweet potato, raw	5" diameter	.1	1.2	0
Sweet potato, baked	½ cup	0.0	.9	0
Sweet potato, canned, syrup, solid+liquid	½ cup	.1	.6	0
Taro, raw	½ cup	0.0	.6	0
Taro, cooked	½ cup	0.0	0.0	0
Tomatillos, raw	½ cup	0.0	.4	0
Tomato, red, ripe, raw	2⅗" diameter	.1	.4	0
Tomato, red, ripe, boiled	½ cup	.1	.4	0
Tomato, canned, whole	½ cup	0.0	.4	0
Tomato, canned, stewed	½ cup	0.0	0.0	0
Tomato, wedges, canned	½ cup	0.0	0.0	0
Tomato juice	½ cup	0.0	.2	0
Tomato paste, canned	½ cup	.2	1.7	0
Tomato puree, canned	½ cup	0.0	.9	0
Tomatoes, sun-dried	1 cup	.2	2.0	0
Tomatoes, sun-dried, oil-packed	1 cup	2.1	0.0	0
Turnips, raw	½ cup	0.0	.4	0
Turnips, boiled	½ cup	0.0	.5	0
Turnip greens, raw	½ cup	0.0	.2	0

Food	Portion	SF1	SF2	Chol
Turnip greens, boiled	½ cup	0.0	.7	0
Vegetable juice cocktail	½ cup	0.0	.3	0
Water chestnut, Chinese, raw	½ cup	0.0	.6	0
Water chestnut, canned, solid+liquid	½ cup	0.0	.5	0
Watercress, raw	½ cup	0.0	.1	0
Waxgourd, raw	½ cup	0.0	.6	0
Waxgourd, boiled	½ cup	0.0	.3	0
Yam, raw	½ cup	0.0	.9	0
Yam, boiled/baked	½ cup	0.0	.8	0

BEANS AND LEGUMES

Food	Portion	SF1	SF2	Chol
Adzuki, cooked	½ cup	0.0	0.0	0
Baked, canned, plain	½ cup	.1	1.9	0
Baked, canned, with beef	½ cup	2.2	0.0	29
Baked, canned, with franks	½ cup	3.0	2.6	8
Baked, canned, with pork	½ cup	.8	2.1	9
Black, cooked	½ cup	.1	2.2	0
Cranberry, cooked	½ cup	.1	0.0	0
French, cooked	½ cup	.1	0.0	0
Great Northern, cooked	½ cup	.1	1.8	0
Kidney, all, cooked	½ cup	.1	3.0	0
Kidney, canned	½ cup	.1	0.0	0
Navy, cooked	½ cup	.1	0.0	0
Pink, cooked	½ cup	.1	1.3	0
Pinto, cooked	½ cup	.1	2.0	0
Pinto, canned	½ cup	.1	1.3	0
Small white, cooked	½ cup	.1	0.0	0
Yardlong, cooked	½ cup	.1	0.0	0
Yellow, cooked	½ cup	.2	0.0	0
White, cooked	½ cup	.1	1.5	0
Winged, cooked	½ cup	.7	0.0	0
Broadbean, cooked	½ cup	.1	1.4	0
Chickpea, cooked	½ cup	.2	1.5	0
Cowpea, catjang, cooked	½ cup	.2	0.0	0
Cowpea, cooked	½ cup	.1	1.7	0
Falafel	1 patty, 2¼"	.4	0.0	0

Food	Portion	SF1	SF2	Chol
Hummus	½ cup	3.1	3.8	0
Hyacinth, cooked	½ cup	.1	0.0	0
Lentils, cooked	½ cup	0.0	1.0	0
Lima, cooked	½ cup	.1	1.0	0
Lupin, cooked	½ cup	.3	.7	0
Miso	½ cup	1.2	2.2	0
Mothbeans, cooked	½ cup	.1	0.0	0
Mung, cooked	½ cup	.1	2.3	0
Mungo, cooked	½ cup	0.0	1.7	0
Natto	½ cup	1.4	1.4	0
Peas, split, cooked	½ cup	.1	1.5	0
Pigeon peas, cooked	½ cup	.1	0.0	0
Refried beans, canned	½ cup	.5	2.0	0
Soybeans, cooked	½ cup	1.1	1.5	0
Soybeans, dry roasted	½ cup	2.7	2.1	0
Soybeans, roasted	½ cup	3.2	0.0	0
Soy milk, fluid	1 cup	.5	.9	0
Tempeh	½ cup	.9	0.0	0
Tofu, raw, firm, nigari	½ cup	1.6	.9	0
Tofu, raw, regular, nigari	½ cup	.9	.4	0
Tofu, dried-frozen, nigari	½ cup	4.4	0.0	0
Tofu, fried, nigari	½ cup	2.9	1.2	0
Tofu, okara, nigari	½ cup	.1	0.0	0

FRUITS & FRUIT JUICES

Food	Portion	SF1	SF2	Chol
Acerola, raw	1 fruit	0.0	0.0	0
Acerola juice, raw	1 cup	0.0	.2	0
Apple, raw, with skin	1 fruit, 5 oz.	.1	1.1	0
Apple, raw, no skin	1 fruit, 5 oz.	.1	.7	0
Apple, dehydrated	1 cup	.1	2.2	0
Apple, dried, cooked, no sugar	1 cup	0.0	1.5	0
Apple juice, canned	1 cup	0.0	.4	0
Apple juice, frozen, diluted	1 cup	0.0	.4	0
Applesauce, canned, unsweetened	1 cup	0.0	2.0	0
Apricots, raw	3 fruits, 4 oz.	0.0	1.0	0

Food	Portion	SF1	SF2	Chol
Apricots, canned, with water+skin	1 cup halves	0.0	.9	0
Apricots, canned, with water, no skin	1 cup whole, no pits	0.0	0.0	0
Apricots, canned, with juice+skin	1 cup halves	0.0	1.0	0
Apricots, dehydrated	1 cup	.1	0.0	0
Apricots, dried	1 cup halves	0.0	3.5	0
Apricots, dried, cooked, no sugar	1 cup halves	0.0	2.6	0
Apricots, frozen, sweetened	1 cup	0.0	1.2	0
Apricot nectar, canned	1 cup	0.0	.5	0
Avocado, raw, all varieties	1 fruit, no skin/seeds	4.9	3.6	0
Banana, raw	1 fruit	.2	.5	0
Blackberries, raw	1 cup	0.0	2.2	0
Blackberries, canned, heavy syrup	1 cup	0.0	2.6	0
Blackberries, frozen, unsweetened	1 cup	0.0	2.3	0
Blueberries, raw	1 cup	0.2	1.0	0
Blueberries, canned, heavy syrup	1 cup	0.0	.6	0
Blueberries, frozen, unsweetened	1 cup	0.0	.6	0
Boysenberries, canned, heavy syrup	1 cup	0.0	2.0	0
Boysenberries, frozen, unsweetened	1 cup	0.0	2.0	0
Breadfruit, raw	1 cup	0.0	3.2	0
Carambola, raw	1 cup	0.0	1.1	0
Carissa, raw	1 cup	0.0	0.0	0
Cherimoya, raw	1 cup	0.0	1.4	0
Cherry, sour, red, raw	1 cup, no pits	.1	.6	0
Cherry, sour, canned, with water	1 cup	.1	.6	0
Cherry, sour, frozen, unsweetened	1 cup	.2	.6	0
Cherry, sweet, raw	1 cup	.3	1.0	0
Cherry, sweet, canned, with water	1 cup	.1	.5	0

Food	Portion	SF1	SF2	Chol
Cherry, sweet, frozen, sweetened	1 cup	.1	.8	0
Coconut, dried, unsweetened	1 cup	114.4	10.0	0
Coconut, dried, sweet, flakes	1 cup	24.0	.8	0
Coconut, dried, toasted	1 cup	83.4	0.0	0
Coconut cream, canned	1 cup	46.5	2.0	0
Coconut cream, raw	1 cup	73.8	0.0	0
Coconut milk, canned	1 cup	42.7	0.0	0
Coconut milk, raw	1 cup	50.7	1.6	0
Coconut water	1 cup	.4	.8	0
Crabapple, raw	1 cup, with skin	.1	0.0	0
Cranberries, raw	1 cup, whole	0.0	1.2	0
Cranberry juice cocktail, bottled	1 cup	0.0	0.0	0
Cranberry sauce, canned, sweetened	1 cup	0.0	.8	0
Currants, black, raw	1 cup	0.0	0.0	0
Currants, red/white, raw	1 cup	0.0	1.4	0
Currants, zante, dried	1 cup	0.0	2.9	0
Custard-apple, raw	1 cup	0.0	0.0	0
Dates, domestic, dry	1 cup	0.0	2.6	0
Elderberries, raw	1 cup	0.0	3.0	0
Fig, raw	1 medium	0.1	1.0	0
Figs, canned	1 cup	0.0	1.6	0
Figs, dried, raw	1 cup	.5	5.6	0
Figs, dried, cooked	1 cup	.3	3.7	0
Fruit cocktail, canned	1 cup	0.0	.8	0
Gooseberries, raw	1 cup	.1	1.9	0
Gooseberries, canned, light syrup	1 cup	0.0	1.8	0
Grapefruit, all	½ fruit, 3.75" diameter	0.0	.5	0
Grapefruit juice, canned	1 cup	0.0	.1	0
Grapefruit juice, frozen, diluted	1 cup	0 0	1	0
Grapefruit juice, white, fresh	1 cup	0.0	1	0
Grapes, raw	1 cup	1	.2	0

Food	Portion	SF1	SF2	Chol
Grape juice, canned/bottled	1 cup	.1	.1	0
Grape juice, frozen, sweetened, diluted	1 cup	.1	.1	0
Ground cherries, raw	1 cup	0.0	0.0	0
Guavas, raw, common	1 cup	.3	2.7	0
Guavas, raw, strawberry	1 cup	.4	0.0	0
Jackfruit, raw	1 cup	0.0	1.0	0
Java-plum, raw	1 cup	0.0	0.0	0
Jujube	1 cup	0.0	0.0	0
Kiwi fruit, raw	1 medium	0.0	.8	0
Kumquat, raw	1 fruit	0.0	.4	0
Lemon, raw, no peel	1 medium	0.0	.5	0
Lemon juice, raw	1 tbsp.	0.0	0.0	0
Lemon juice, canned/bottled	1 tbsp.	0.0	0.0	0
Lemon juice, frozen, unconcentrated	1 tbsp.	0.0	0.0	0
Lemon peel, raw	1 tbsp.	0.0	.2	0
Lime, raw	1 fruit, 2" diameter	0.0	.6	0
Lime juice, raw	1 tbsp.	0.0	0.0	0
Lime juice, canned/bottled	1 tbsp.	0.0	0.0	0
Lychee, raw	1 cup	0.0	.7	0
Lychee, dried	1 cup	0.0	2.8	0
Loganberries, frozen	1 cup	0.0	2.2	0
Longans, raw	1 cup	0.0	.6	0
Longans, dried	1 cup	0.0	0.0	0
Loquat, raw	1 fruit	0.0	.1	0
Mammy-apple, raw	1 fruit	0.0	7.6	0
Mango, raw	1 fruit	.1	1.1	0
Melon, cantaloupe, raw	½ fruit	0.1	.6	0
Melon, casaba, raw	1/10 fruit	0.0	.4	0
Melon, honeydew, raw	1/10 fruit	0.0	.2	0
Mullberries, raw	1 cup	0.0	.7	0
Nectarine, raw	1 fruit	0.1	.5	0
Oheloberries, raw	1 cup	0.0	0.0	0
Olives, ripe, canned	1 small	0.0	0.0	0
	1 large	1	0 0	0
	1 jumbo	1	0 0	0
Orange, raw, all varieties	1 fruit, 2⅝" diameter	0.0	7	0

COUNT OUT CHOLESTEROL

Food	Portion	SF1	SF2	Chol
Orange juice, raw	1 cup	.1	.3	0
Orange juice, canned	1 cup	0.0	.1	0
Orange juice, frozen, with water	1 cup	0.0	.1	0
Orange peel, raw	1 tbsp.	0.0	.1	0
Papaya, raw	1 fruit, 3½" diameter	.1	1.6	0
Papaya nectar, canned	1 cup	.1	.5	0
Passion-fruit, purple, raw	1 fruit	0.0	.6	0
Passion-fruit juice, purple, raw	1 cup	0.0	.1	0
Peach, raw	1 fruit, 4/pound	0.0	.5	0
Peaches, canned	1 cup	0.0	.7	0
Peaches, dehydrated	1 cup	.1	0.0	0
Peaches, dried	1 cup	.1	3.9	0
Peaches, frozen, sweetened	1 cup	0.0	1.1	0
Peach nectar, canned	1 cup	0.0	.4	0
Pear, raw	1 fruit, 2.5/pound	0.0	1.0	0
Pears, canned	1 cup	0.0	1.5	0
Pears, dried	1 cup	.1	4.1	0
Pear nectar, canned	1 cup	0.0	.5	0
Persimmon, Japan, raw	1 fruit, 2½" diameter	0.0	1.8	0
Persimmon, Japan, dried	1 cup	0.0	8.8	0
Persimmon, native, raw	1 fruit	0.0	0.0	0
Pineapple, raw	1 slice, 3½" diameter	0.0	.3	0
Pineapple, canned	1 cup tidbits	0.0	.5	0
Pineapple, frozen	1 cup chunks	0.0	.8	0
Pineapple juice, canned	1 cup	0.0	.1	0
Pineapple juice, frozen, with water	1 cup	0.0	.1	0
Pitanga, raw	1 fruit	0.0	0.0	0
Plantain, raw	1 fruit	0.0	1.2	0
Plantain, cooked	1 cup	0.0	1.1	0
Plum, raw	1 fruit, 2⅛" diameter	0.0	.3	0
Plums, purple, canned	1 cup	0.0	.7	0

Food	Portion	SF1	SF2	Chol
Pomegranate, raw	1 fruit, 3⅜" diameter	0.0	.3	0
Pricklypear, raw	1 fruit	0.0	1.1	0
Prunes, canned, heavy syrup	1 cup	0.0	2.7	0
Prunes, dehydrated	1 cup	.1	0.0	0
Prunes, dried	1 cup, no pits	.1	3.4	0
Prune juice, canned	1 cup	0.0	.8	0
Pummelo, raw	1 fruit	0.0	1.8	0
Quince, raw	1 fruit	0.0	.5	0
Raisins, seeded	1 cup	.3	3.0	0
Raisins, seedless	1 cup	.4	2.8	0
Raspberries, raw	1 cup	0.0	2.5	0
Raspberries, red, frozen	1 cup	0.0	3.3	0
Rhubarb, raw	1 cup	0.0	.7	0
Rhubarb, frozen, raw	1 cup	0.0	.7	0
Rhubarb, frozen, cooked, with sugar	1 cup	0.0	1.4	0
Sapodilla, raw	1 fruit, 3" diameter	0.0	2.7	0
Sapotes, raw	1 fruit	0.0	1.8	0
Soursop, raw	1 fruit	0.0	6.2	0
Strawberries, raw	1 cup	0.0	1.0	0
Strawberries, frozen, no sugar	1 cup, unthawed	0.0	.9	0
Strawberries, frozen, sweetened, whole	1 cup	0.0	1.5	0
Sugar-apple, raw	1 fruit, 2⅞" diameter	0.0	2.0	0
Tamarind, raw	1 fruit, 3" x 1"	0.0	0.0	0
Tangerine, raw	1 fruit, 2⅜" diameter	0.0	.6	0
Tangerines, canned, with juice	1 cup	0.0	.5	0
Tangerine juice, raw	1 cup	.1	.1	0
Tangerine juice, frozen, sweetened, diluted	1 cup	0.0	0.0	0
Watermelon, raw	1/16 fruit, 10" diameter	0.0	.7	0

POULTRY

Food	Portion	SF1	SF2	Chol
Chicken, fresh				
White, with skin, fried	4 oz.	4.8	0.0	100
White, with skin, roasted	4 oz.	3.4	0.0	96
Dark, with skin, fried	4 oz.	8.1	0.0	104
Dark, with skin, roasted	4 oz.	5.0	0.0	104
Light, no skin, roasted	4 oz.	1.3	0.0	86
Dark, no skin, roasted	4 oz.	3.1	0.0	106
Breast, with skin, roasted	4 oz.	3.4	0.0	96
Breast, no skin, roasted	4 oz.	1.3	0.0	86
Drumstick, with skin, roasted	4 oz.	5.0	0.0	104
Drumstick, no skin, roasted	4 oz.	3.1	0.0	106
Leg, with skin, roasted	4 oz.	5.0	0.0	104
Leg, no skin, roasted	4 oz.	3.1	0.0	106
Thigh, with skin, roasted	4 oz.	5.0	0.0	104
Thigh, no skin, roasted	4 oz.	3.1	0.0	106
Wing, with skin, roasted	4 oz.	5.0	0.0	104
Wing, no skin, roasted	4 oz.	3.1	0.0	106
Chicken frankfurter	1 oz.	2.5	0.0	45
Chicken roll, white	2 oz.	1.1	0.0	28
Turkey, fresh				
White, with skin, roasted	4 oz.	1.5	0.0	108
Dark, with skin, roasted	4 oz.	2.4	0.0	134
White, no skin, roasted	4 oz.	.5	0.0	100
Dark, no skin, roasted	4 oz.	1.6	0.0	128
Breast, with skin, roasted	4 oz.	1.5	0.0	108
Leg, with skin, roasted	4 oz.	2.4	0.0	134
Wing, with skin, roasted	4 oz.	2.4	0.0	134
Turkey bologna	2 oz.	2.9	0.0	20
Turkey frankfurter	1 oz.	2.8	0.0	40
Turkey, with gravy, frozen	5 oz.	1.2	0.0	26
Turkey, ground, cooked	4 oz.	2.8	0.0	84
Turkey roll, light	2 oz.	.1	0.0	24
Duck, no skin, roasted	4 oz.	4.8	0.0	103
Goose liver pâté	1 oz.	4.1	0.0	43

SEAFOOD

Food	Portion	SF1	SF2	Chol
Abalone, raw	3 oz.	.1	0.0	72
Abalone, fried	3 oz.	1.4	0.0	80
Anchovies, canned, with oil, drained	5 anchovies	.4	0.0	17
Bass, cooked, dry	3 oz.	.9	0.0	74
Bass, stripe, cooked, dry heat	3 oz.	.6	0.0	88
Bluefish, cooked, dry	3 oz.	1.0	0.0	65
Burbot, cooked, dry	3 oz.	.2	0.0	65
Butterfish, cooked, dry	3 oz.	0.0	0.0	71
Carp, baked/broiled	3 oz.	1.2	0.0	71
Catfish, breaded+fried	3 oz.	2.8	0.0	69
Catfish, farmed, cooked, dry heat	3 oz.	1.5	0.0	54
Catfish, wild, cooked, dry heat	3 oz.	.6	0.0	61
Caviar, black/red	1 oz.	1.1	0.0	165
Cisco, smoked	3 oz.	1.5	0.0	27
Clam, raw	3 oz.	.1	0.0	29
Clam, boiled/steamed	3 oz.	.2	0.0	60
Clam, breaded+fried	3 oz.	2.3	0.0	52
Clam, canned, drained	3 oz.	.2	0.0	57
Clam, canned, with liquid	3 oz.	0.0	0.0	3
Cod, Atlantic, baked/broiled	3 oz.	.2	0.0	51
Cod, Atlantic, canned, solid+liquid	3 oz.	.1	0.0	47
Cod, Atlantic, dried+salted	3 oz.	.4	0.0	129
Cod, Pacific, cooked, dry	3 oz.	.1	0.0	40
Crab, Alaska king, raw	3 oz.	.1	0.0	36
Crab, blue, raw	3 oz.	.2	0.0	66
Crab, blue, boiled/steamed	3 oz.	.2	0.0	86
Crab, blue, canned	3 oz.	.2	0.0	76
Crab, blue, cakes	3 oz.	1.1	0.0	112
Crab, dungeness, raw	3 oz.	.1	0.0	50
Crab, dungeness, cooked, moist heat	3 oz.	.1	0.0	65
Crab, king, boiled/steamed	3 oz.	.1	0.0	45
Crab, king, imitation	3 oz.	.2	0.0	17

Food	Portion	SF1	SF2	Chol
Crab, queen, raw	3 oz.	.1	0.0	47
Crab, queen, cooked, moist heat	3 oz.	.2	0.0	60
Crayfish, wild, raw	3 oz.	.1	0.0	97
Crayfish, wild, cooked, moist heat	3 oz.	.2	0.0	113
Crayfish, farmed, cooked, moist heat	3 oz.	.2	0.0	116
Croaker, Atlantic, breaded+fried	3 oz.	3.0	0.0	71
Cusk, cooked, dry	3 oz.	0.0	0.0	45
Cuttlefish, raw	3 oz.	.1	0.0	95
Cuttlefish, cooked	3 oz.	.2	0.0	190
Drum, freshwater, cooked, dry	3 oz.	1.2	0.0	70
Eel, raw	3 oz.	2.0	0.0	107
Eel, baked/broiled	3 oz.	2.6	0.0	137
Fish sticks, frozen, reheated	1 stick	.9	0.0	31
Flatfish, baked/broiled	3 oz.	.3	0.0	58
Gefilte fish, sweet	3 oz.	.3	0.0	23
Grouper, baked/broiled	3 oz.	.3	0.0	43
Haddock, baked/broiled	3 oz.	.2	0.0	60
Haddock, smoked	3 oz.	.1	0.0	65
Halibut, baked/broiled	3 oz.	.4	0.0	34
Halibut, Greenland, raw	3 oz.	2.1	0.0	39
Halibut, Greenland, cooked, dry	3 oz.	2.6	0.0	50
Herring, Atlantic, baked/broiled	3 oz.	2.2	0.0	65
Herring, Atlantic, pickled	3 oz.	1.8	0.0	10
Herring, Atlantic, kippered	3 oz.	2.1	0.0	62
Herring, Pacific, cooked, dry	3 oz.	3.5	0.0	84
Ling, cooked, dry	3 oz.	0.0	0.0	43
Lingcod, cooked, dry	3 oz.	.2	0.0	57
Lobster, northern, raw	3 oz.	.2	0.0	81
Lobster, northern, boiled/steamed	3 oz.	.1	0.0	61
Lobster, spiny, cooked, moist heat	3 oz.	.3	0.0	77

Food	Portion	SF1	SF2	Chol
Mackerel, cooked	3 oz.	2.4	0.0	51
Mackerel, canned, dry, solid	1 cup	3.5	0.0	150
Mackerel, Atlantic, baked/broiled	3 oz.	3.5	0.0	64
Mackerel, king, cooked, dry	3 oz.	.4	0.0	58
Milkfish, cooked, dry	3 oz.	0.0	0.0	57
Monkfish, cooked, dry	3 oz.	0.0	0.0	27
Mullet, striped, baked/broiled	3 oz.	1.2	0.0	54
Mussels, blue, raw	3 oz.	.4	0.0	24
Mussels, blue, boiled/steamed	3 oz.	.7	0.0	51
Ocean Perch, baked/broiled	3 oz.	.3	0.0	46
Octopus, common, raw	3 oz.	.2	0.0	41
Octopus, common, cooked, moist	3 oz.	.4	0.0	82
Orange Roughy, cooked, dry	3 oz.	0.0	0.0	22
Oyster, east, farmed, raw	3 oz.	.4	0.0	21
Oyster, east, farmed, cooked, dry heat	3 oz.	.6	0.0	32
Oyster, east, wild, raw	3 oz.	.7	0.0	49
Oyster, east, wild, cooked, dry heat	3 oz.	.5	0.0	42
Oyster, east, wild, cooked, moist heat	3 oz.	1.3	0.0	94
Oyster, east, canned	3 oz.	.5	0.0	47
Oyster, Pacific, raw	3 oz.	.4	0.0	43
Oyster, Pacific, cooked, moist heat	3 oz.	.9	0.0	85
Perch, baked/broiled	3 oz.	.2	0.0	34
Pike, north, baked/broiled	3 oz.	.1	0.0	43
Pike, walleye, cooked, dry	3 oz.	.3	0.0	94
Pollock, Atlantic, cooked, dry	3 oz.	.1	0.0	77
Pollock, walleye, baked/broiled	3 oz.	.2	0.0	86
Pompano, baked/broiled	3 oz.	3.8	0.0	54
Pout, ocean, cooked, dry	3 oz.	.3	0.0	57
Rockfish, baked/broiled	3 oz.	.4	0.0	34

Food	Portion	SF1	SF2	Chol
Roe, raw	3 oz.	1.2	0.0	318
Roe, mixed, cooked, dry	3 oz.	1.6	0.0	407
Sablefish, cooked, dry	3 oz.	3.5	0.0	54
Sablefish, smoked	3 oz.	3.6	0.0	54
Salmon, Atlantic, farmed, raw	3 oz.	1.9	0.0	50
Salmon, Atlantic, farmed, cooked, dry heat	3 oz.	2.1	0.0	54
Salmon, Atlantic, wild, cooked, dry heat	3 oz.	1.1	0.0	60
Salmon, chinook, smoked, lox	3 oz.	.8	0.0	20
Salmon, chinook, cooked, dry	3 oz.	2.7	0.0	72
Salmon, chum, cooked, dry	3 oz.	.9	0.0	81
Salmon, chum, canned, drained	3 oz.	1.3	0.0	33
Salmon, coho, farmed, raw	3 oz.	1.5	0.0	43
Salmon, coho, farmed, cooked, dry heat	3 oz.	1.7	0.0	54
Salmon, coho, wild, cooked, moist heat	3 oz.	1.4	0.0	48
Salmon, coho, wild, cooked, dry heat	3 oz.	.9	0.0	47
Salmon, pink, canned, solid+liquid	3 oz.	1.3	0.0	47
Salmon, pink, cooked, dry	3 oz.	.6	0.0	57
Salmon, sockeye, raw	3 oz.	1.3	0.0	53
Salmon, sockeye, baked/broiled	3 oz.	1.6	0.0	74
Salmon, sockeye, canned, drained	3 oz.	1.4	0.0	37
Sardines, canned, oil, drained	2 sardines	.4	0.0	34
Sardines, canned, with tomato sauce, drained	1 sardine	1.2	.1	23
Scallop, raw	3 oz.	.1	0.0	28
Scallop, breaded+fried	3 oz.	2.7	0.0	61
Scallop, imitation	3 oz.	.1	0.0	19

Food	Portion	SF1	SF2	Chol
Scup, cooked, dry	3 oz.	0.0	0.0	57
Sea bass, baked/broiled	3 oz.	.5	0.0	43
Sea trout, mixed, cooked, dry	3 oz.	1.1	0.0	90
Shad, American, cooked, dry	3 oz.	0.0	0.0	82
Shark, raw	3 oz.	.8	0.0	43
Shark, battered+fried	3 oz.	2.7	0.0	50
Sheepshead, baked/broiled	3 oz.	.3	0.0	54
Shrimp, raw	3 oz.	.3	0.0	129
Shrimp, boiled/steamed	3 oz.	.3	0.0	171
Shrimp, breaded+fried	3 oz.	1.8	0.0	150
Shrimp, canned	3 oz.	.3	0.0	147
Shrimp, imitation	3 oz.	.2	0.0	31
Smelt, rainbow, baked/broiled	3 oz.	.5	0.0	77
Snapper, baked/broiled	3 oz.	.3	0.0	43
Spot, cooked, dry	3 oz.	1.6	0.0	65
Squid, raw	3 oz.	.3	0.0	198
Squid, fried	3 oz.	1.6	0.0	221
Sturgeon, baked/broiled	3 oz.	1.0	0.0	65
Sturgeon, smoked	3 oz.	.9	0.0	68
Sucker, white, cooked, dry	3 oz.	.5	0.0	45
Sunfish, cooked, dry	3 oz.	.2	0.0	73
Surimi	3 oz.	.2	0.0	26
Swordfish, baked/broiled	3 oz.	1.2	0.0	43
Tilefish, baked/broiled	3 oz.	.7	0.0	54
Trout, rainbow, farmed, raw	3 oz.	1.3	0.0	50
Trout, rainbow, farmed, cooked, dry heat	3 oz.	1.8	0.0	58
Trout, rainbow, wild, cooked, dry heat	3 oz.	1.0	0.0	60
Trout, mixed, cooked, dry	3 oz.	1.3	0.0	63
Tuna, bluefin, baked/broiled	3 oz.	1.3	0.0	43
Tuna, light, canned, oil, drained	3 oz.	1.3	0.0	15
Tuna, light, canned, water, drained	3 oz.	1.2	0.0	26

Food	Portion	SF1	SF2	Chol
Tuna, white, canned, oil, drained	3 oz.	1.4	0.0	26
Tuna, white, canned, water, drained	3 oz.	.6	0.0	36
Tuna, skipjack, cooked, dry	3 oz.	.4	0.0	51
Tuna, yellowfin, cooked, dry	3 oz.	.3	0.0	49
Turbot, European, cooked, dry	3 oz.	0.0	0.0	53
Whelk, raw	3 oz.	0.0	0.0	55
Whelk, boiled/steamed	3 oz.	.1	0.0	111
Whitefish, smoked	3 oz.	.2	0.0	28
Whitefish, mixed, cooked, dry	3 oz.	1.0	0.0	65
Whiting, baked/broiled	3 oz.	.3	0.0	71
Wolffish, Atlantic, cooked, dry	3 oz.	.4	0.0	50
Yellowtail, mixed, cooked, dry	3 oz.	0.0	0.0	60

BEEF

Food	Portion	SF1	SF2	Chol
Arm, lean+fat, braised	3 oz.	8.6	0.0	84
Arm, lean, braised	3 oz.	2.9	0.0	86
Blade, lean+fat, braised	3 oz.	8.7	0.0	88
Blade, lean, braised	3 oz.	4.3	0.0	90
Bottom round, lean+fat, braised	3 oz.	5.4	0.0	82
Bottom round, lean, braised	3 oz	2.4	0.0	82
Brain, simmered	3 oz.	2.5	0.0	1746
Brisket, flat, lean+fat, braised	3 oz.	9.4	0.0	81
Brisket, flat, lean, braised	3 oz.	2.7	0.0	81
Brisket, point, lean+fat, braised	3 oz.	11.5	0.0	78
Brisket, point, lean, braised	3 oz.	5.0	0.0	77
Eye of round, lean+fat, roasted	3 oz.	4.2	0.0	61

Food	Portion	SF1	SF2	Chol
Eye of round, lean, roasted	3 oz.	1.5	0.0	59
Ground, lean, broiled	3 oz.	6.0	0.0	77
Ground, regular, broiled	3 oz.	6.5	0.0	86
Heart, simmered	3 oz.	1.4	0.0	164
Kidney, simmered	3 oz.	.9	0.0	329
Liver, braised	3 oz.	1.6	0.0	331
Liver, pan fried	3 oz.	2.3	0.0	410
Patty, frozen, broiled	3 oz.	6.6	0.0	80
Porterhouse, lean+fat, broiled	3 oz.	7.6	0.0	71
Porterhouse, lean, broiled	3 oz.	3.7	0.0	68
Rib, large, lean+fat, broiled	3 oz.	9.8	0.0	80
Rib, large, lean, broiled	3 oz.	6.0	0.0	77
Rib, small, lean+fat, roasted	3 oz.	9.6	0.0	71
Rib, small, lean, roasted	3 oz.	3.5	0.0	67
Round, lean+fat, broiled	3 oz.	4.4	0.0	68
Round, lean, broiled	3 oz.	2.2	0.0	66
Shank, lean+fat, simmered	3 oz.	4.8	0.0	68
Shank, lean, simmered	3 oz.	1.9	0.0	66
Shortrib, lean+fat, braised	3 oz.	15.1	0.0	80
Shortrib, lean, braised	3 oz.	6.6	0.0	79
Sirloin, lean+fat, broiled	3 oz.	5.2	0.0	78
Sirloin, lean, broiled	3 oz.	3.3	0.0	77
T-bone, lean+fat, broiled	3 oz.	7.3	0.0	71
T-bone, lean, broiled	3 oz.	3.3	0.0	68
Tenderloin, lean+fat, broiled	3 oz.	6.8	0.0	71
Tenderloin, lean, broiled	3 oz.	3.3	0.0	68
Tip round, lean+fat, roasted	3 oz.	4.3	0.0	70
Tip round, lean, roasted	3 oz.	2.0	0.0	69
Tongue, simmered	3 oz.	7.6	0.0	91
Toploin, lean+fat, broiled	3 oz.	6.6	0.0	67
Toploin, lean, broiled	3 oz.	3.1	0.0	65
Top round, lean+fat, broiled	3 oz.	3.1	0.0	72
Top round, lean, broiled	3 oz.	1.4	0.0	71

Food	Portion	SF1	SF2	Chol
Breakfast strip, cooked	3 oz.	12.2	0.0	101
Corned beef brisket, canned	3 oz.	5.4	0.0	72
Corned beef brisket, cooked	3 oz.	5.6	0.0	86
Dried beef, cured	3 oz.	1.5	0.0	36
Sausage, cooked, smoked	1 oz.	3.3	0.0	20

LAMB

Food	Portion	SF1	SF2	Chol
Brain, braised	3 oz.	2.2	0.0	1737
Ground, broiled	3 oz.	6.9	0.0	82
Heart, braised	3 oz.	2.7	0.0	212
Kidney, braised	3 oz.	1.0	0.0	480
Leg, lean+fat, cooked	3 oz.	6.5	0.0	86
Leg, lean, cooked	3 oz.	2.6	0.0	77
Liver, braised	3 oz.	2.9	0.0	426
Liver, pan-fried	3 oz.	4.2	0.0	419
Loin, lean+fat, broiled	3 oz.	10.2	0.0	95
Loin, lean, broiled	3 oz.	3.0	0.0	97
Rib, lean+fat, roasted	3 oz.	12.3	0.0	90
Rib, lean, roasted	3 oz.	4.2	0.0	94
Shank, lean+fat, cooked	3 oz.	6.6	0.0	87
Shank, lean, cooked	3 oz.	2.2	0.0	86
Shoulder, lean+fat, braised	3 oz.	10.8	0.0	105
Shoulder, lean, braised	3 oz.	5.8	0.0	108

VEAL

Food	Portion	SF1	SF2	Chol
Arm, lean+fat, roasted	3 oz.	3.0	0.0	92
Arm, lean, roasted	3 oz.	2.0	0.0	93
Blade, lean+fat, roasted	3 oz.	2.9	0.0	99
Blade, lean, roasted	3 oz.	2.2	0.0	101
Brain, braised	3 oz.	1.9	0.0	2635
Ground, broiled	3 oz.	2.6	0.0	88
Heart, braised	3 oz.	1.5	0.0	150
Kidney, braised	3 oz.	1.5	0.0	672
Leg, lean+fat, roasted	3 oz.	1.6	0.0	88

Food	Portion	SF1	SF2	Chol
Leg, lean, roasted	3 oz.	1.0	0.0	88
Liver, braised	3 oz.	2.2	0.0	477
Liver, pan-fried	3 oz.	3.6	0.0	281
Loin, lean+fat, roasted	3 oz.	4.5	0.0	88
Loin, lean, roasted	3 oz.	2.2	0.0	90
Rib, lean+fat, roasted	3 oz.	4.3	0.0	111
Rib, lean, roasted	3 oz.	1.8	0.0	112
Shoulder, lean+fat, roasted	3 oz.	2.9	0.0	96
Shoulder, lean, roasted	3 oz.	2.1	0.0	97
Sirloin, lean+fat, roasted	3 oz.	3.8	0.0	87
Sirloin, lean, roasted	3 oz.	2.0	0.0	88

PORK

Food	Portion	SF1	SF2	Chol
Blade, lean & fat, roasted	3 oz.	7.8	0.0	79
Blade, lean, roasted	3 oz.	4.5	0.0	79
Brains, braised	3 oz.	1.8	0.0	2169
Center loin, lean & fat, roasted	3 oz.	4.3	0.0	68
Center loin, lean, roasted	3 oz.	2.8	0.0	67
Center rib, lean & fat, broiled	3 oz.	4.8	0.0	70
Center rib, lean, broiled	3 oz.	2.9	0.0	69
Ground, cooked	3 oz.	6.6	0.0	80
Liver, braised	3 oz.	1.2	0.0	302
Loin, lean & fat, roasted	3 oz.	4.6	0.0	70
Loin, lean, roasted	3 oz.	3.0	0.0	69
Picnic, fresh, lean & fat, roasted	3 oz.	7.5	0.0	80
Picnic, fresh, lean, roasted	3 oz.	3.7	0.0	81
Sirloin, lean & fat, broiled	3 oz.	5.0	0.0	73
Sirloin, lean, broiled	3 oz.	3.1	0.0	72
Sirloin, lean, roasted	3 oz.	3.1	0.0	73
Spare rib, fresh, cooked	3 oz.	10.3	0.0	103
Tenderloin, lean, roasted	3 oz.	1.4	0.0	67
Tongue, fresh, braised	3 oz.	5.5	0.0	124
Whole shoulder, lean & fat, roasted	3 oz.	6.7	0.0	77

Food	Portion	SF1	SF2	Chol
Whole shoulder, lean, roasted	3 oz.	4.1	0.0	77
Ham, fresh, whole leg, lean & fat, roasted	3 oz.	5.5	0.0	80
Ham, fresh, whole leg, lean, roasted	3 oz.	2.8	0.0	80
Ham, fresh, rump, lean & fat, roasted	3 oz.	4.5	0.0	82
Ham, fresh, rump, lean, roasted	3 oz.	2.4	0.0	82
Ham, fresh, shank, lean & fat, roasted	3 oz.	6.3	0.0	78
Ham, fresh, shank, lean, roasted	3 oz.	3.1	0.0	78
Ham patties, grilled	3 oz.	9.2	0.0	59
Ham, cured, lean & fat, roasted	3 oz.	5.1	0.0	53
Ham, cured, lean, roasted	3 oz.	1.6	0.0	47
Bacon, canadian, cooked	3 oz.	2.3	0.0	49
Bacon, cured, cooked	3 oz.	15.0	0.0	78
Bratwurst, cooked	1 oz.	2.6	0.0	17
Chitterlings, cooked	3 oz.	8.6	0.0	122
Pork feet, pickled	1 oz.	1.6	0.0	26
Salt pork, raw	1 oz.	8.3	0.0	24
Sausage, Italian, cooked	4 oz.	7.5	0.0	65
Sausage, fresh, cooked	1 link, 4"	1.5	0.0	10

VARIETY MEATS

Food	Portion	SF1	SF2	Chol
Bacon, fried	1 oz.	5.0	0.0	26
Beef, cured, thin sliced	1 oz.	.5	0.0	12
Bologna, beef	1 oz.	4.0	0.0	16
Bologna, beef/pork	1 oz.	3.0	0.0	20
Bologna, pork	1 oz.	2.0	0.0	17
Bologna, turkey	1 oz.	1.3	0.0	20
Bratwurst, pork, cooked	1 oz.	2.6	0.0	17
Bratwurst, pork/beef	1 oz.	2.8	0.0	18

Food	Portion	SF1	SF2	Chol
Chorizo, pork/beef	1 oz.	4.1	0.0	25
Corned beef loaf, jellied	1 oz.	.7	0.0	13
Dutch brand loaf, pork/beef	1 oz.	1.8	0.0	13
Frankfurter, beef	1 frank	6.0	0.0	30
Frankfurter, beef/pork	1 oz.	3.1	0.0	15
Hamsteak, extra lean, unheated	1 oz.	.4	0.0	13
Ham, canned, extra lean, unheated	1 oz.	.4	0.0	11
Ham, canned, unheated	1 oz.	1.2	0.0	11
Ham, chopped, canned	1 oz.	1.8	0.0	14
Ham, chopped, not canned	1 oz.	1.6	0.0	14
Ham, minced	1 oz.	2.0	0.0	20
Ham, sliced, extra lean	1 oz.	.5	0.0	15
Ham, sliced, lean	1 oz.	1.0	0.0	30
Ham salad spread	1 oz.	1.4	0.0	10
Ham and cheese loaf	1 oz.	2.1	0.0	16
Headcheese, pork	1 oz.	1.4	0.0	23
Honey loaf, pork/beef	1 oz.	.4	0.0	10
Honey roll, 10-15%fat	1 oz.	1.2	0.0	14
Kielbasa, pork/beef	1 oz.	2.8	0.0	19
Knackwurst, pork/beef	1 oz.	2.9	0.0	16
Lebanon bologna, beef	1 oz.	1.7	0.0	20
Liver sausage, liver	1 oz.	3.0	0.0	45
Lunchmeat, beef, sliced	1 oz.	.5	0.0	12
Mortadella, beef/pork	1 oz.	2.7	0.0	16
Olive loaf, pork	1 oz.	1.7	0.0	11
Pastrami, beef	1 oz.	3.0	0.0	26
Pepperoni, pork/beef	1 slice, 1⅜" diameter	.9	0.0	4
Pickle & pimiento loaf	1 oz.	2.2	0.0	10
Polish sausage, pork	1 oz.	2.9	0.0	20
Salami, beef, cooked	1 oz.	2.0	0.0	15
Salami, beef/pork, cooked	1 oz.	2.3	0.0	18
Salami, pork, dry	1 oz.	3.4	0.0	22
Salami, pork/beef, dry	1 oz.	2.0	0.0	15
Salami, turkey, cooked	1 oz.	1.1	0.0	23
Sausage, Italian, pork, cooked	4 oz.	7.5	0.0	65

Food	Portion	SF1	SF2	Chol
Sausage, luncheon, pork/beef	1 oz.	2.2	0.0	18
Sausage, pork, fresh, cooked	1 link, 4"	1.5	0.0	10
Sausage, pork/beef, fresh, cooked	1 link, 4"	5.8	0.0	35
Sausage, Vienna, beef/pork	1 sausage, 2"x ⅞"	1.5	0.0	8

GRAVIES

Food	Portion	SF1	SF2	Chol
Au jus, canned	4 oz.	.1	0.0	1
Au jus, dehydrated	4 oz.	.4	0.0	1
Beef, canned	4 oz.	1.5	0.0	4
Beef, dehydrated	4 oz.	.4	0.0	1
Chicken, canned	4 oz.	1.5	0.0	3
Chicken, dehydrated	4 oz.	.3	0.0	1
Mushroom, canned	4 oz.	.5	.2	0
Mushroom, dehydrated	4 oz.	.3	0.0	1
Onion, dehydrated	4 oz.	.2	.2	0
Pork, dehydrated	4 oz.	.4	0.0	1
Turkey, canned	4 oz.	.5	0.0	3
Turkey, dehydrated	4 oz.	.3	0.0	1

SAUCES

Food	Portion	SF1	SF2	Chol
Barbeque, ready-to-serve	4 oz.	.3	0.0	0
Bearnaise	4 oz.	21.0	0.0	100
Cheese	4 oz.	4.5	0.0	30
Curry, dehydrated	4 oz.	.5	0.0	0
Hollandaise	4 oz.	21.0	0.0	90
Marinara, canned	4 oz.	.6	0.0	0
Mushroom, dehydrated	4 oz.	.2	0.0	0
Spaghetti, canned	4 oz.	.9	1.3	0
Stroganoff, dehydrated	4 oz.	1.7	.1	7
Sweet/sour, dehydrated	4 oz.	0.0	0.0	0
Teriyaki, dehydrated	4 oz.	.3	.6	0
Teriyaki, ready-to-serve	1 oz.	0.0	0.0	0
Tomato, canned	4 oz.	0.0	.5	0

Food	Portion	SF1	SF2	Chol
Tomato with herbs and cheese, canned	4 oz.	.8	0.0	0
Tomato with mushrooms, canned	4 oz.	0.0	0.0	0
Tomato with mushrooms and peppers, canned	4 oz.	.2	1.2	0
Tomato with onion, canned	4 oz.	0.0	0.0	0
Tomato with tomato bits, canned	4 oz.	.1	0.0	0
Soy	1 oz.	0.0	0.0	0
Sour cream, dehydrated	4 oz.	6.0	0.0	28
White	4 oz.	3.0	0.0	20

CONDIMENTS

Food	Portion	SF1	SF2	Chol
Catsup	1 tbsp.	0.0	.1	0
Pickle, cucumber, dill	1 medium	0.0	.2	0
Pickle, cucumber, sweet	1 medium	0.0	.1	0
Pickle, cucumber, sour	1 medium	0.0	.1	0
Pimiento, canned	1 tbsp.	0.0	0.0	0
Pickle relish, hamburger	1 tbsp.	0.0	.1	0
Pickle relish, hot dog	1 tbsp.	0.0	0.0	0
Pickle relish, sweet	1 tbsp.	0.0	0.0	0

FATS & OILS

Food	Portion	SF1	SF2	Chol
Fat, chicken	1 tbsp.	3.8	0.0	11
Fat, lard, pork	1 cup	80.4	0.0	164
Margarine, hard, corn	1 tbsp.	2.2	0.0	0
Margarine, hard, safflower	1 tbsp.	1.8	0.0	0
Margarine, hard, soy	1 tbsp.	2.4	0.0	0
Margarine, soft, corn	1 tbsp.	2.1	0.0	0
Margarine, soft, safflower	1 tbsp.	1.8	0.0	0
Margarine, soft, soy	1 tbsp.	1.8	0.0	0
Margarine, liquid, soy	1 tbsp.	1.8	0.0	0
Margarine, spread, tub	1 tbsp.	1.6	0.0	0

COUNT OUT CHOLESTEROL

Food	Portion	SF1	SF2	Chol
Margarine, imitation, corn	1 tbsp.	.9	0.0	0
Margarine, imitation, soy	1 tbsp.	.7	0.0	0
Mayonnaise, soybean	1 tbsp.	1.6	0.0	8
Mayonnaise, safflower/soy	1 tbsp.	1.2	0.0	8
Mayonnaise, imitation, soybean	1 tbsp.	.5	0.0	4
Oil, canola	1 tbsp.	1.0	0.0	0
Oil, vegetable	1 tbsp.	1.6	0.0	0
Oil, vegetable, coconut	1 tbsp.	11.8	0.0	0
Oil, vegetable, corn	1 tbsp.	1.7	0.0	0
Oil, vegetable, cottonseed	1 tbsp.	3.5	0.0	0
Oil, vegetable, olive	1 tbsp.	1.8	0.0	0
Oil, vegetable, palm	1 tbsp.	6.7	0.0	0
Oil, vegetable, peanut	1 tbsp.	2.3	0.0	0
Oil, vegetable, safflower	1 tbsp.	1.0	0.0	0
Oil, vegetable, sesame	1 tbsp.	1.9	0.0	0
Oil, vegetable, soybean	1 tbsp.	2.0	0.0	0
Oil, vegetable, sunflower	1 tbsp.	1.4	0.0	0
Shortening, regular, lard/vegetable	1 tbsp.	5.2	0.0	7
Shortening, regular, soy/cottonseed	1 tbsp.	3.2	0.0	0

SALAD DRESSING

Food	Portion	SF1	SF2	Chol
Blue cheese	1 tbsp.	1.5	0.0	3
French	1 tbsp.	1.5	0.0	1
French, low-cal	1 tbsp.	.1	0.0	1
Italian	1 tbsp.	1.0	0.0	0
Italian, low-cal	1 tbsp.	.2	0.0	1
Mayonnaise-type	1 tbsp.	.7	0.0	4
Russian	1 tbsp.	1.1	0.0	3
Russian, low-cal	1 tbsp.	.1	0.0	1
Sesame seed	1 tbsp.	.9	0.0	0
Thousand Island	1 tbsp.	.9	0.0	4
Thousand Island, low-cal	1 tbsp.	.2	0.0	2
Sandwich spread, unspecified oil	1 tbsp.	.8	0.0	12

HERBS AND SPICES

Food	Portion	SF1	SF2	Chol
Allspice, ground	1 tsp.	0.0	.1	0
Anise seed	1 tsp.	0.0	.1	0
Basil, fresh	5 leaves	0.0	0.0	0
Basil, ground	1 tsp.	0.0	.1	0
Bay leaf, crumbled	1 tsp.	0.0	0.0	0
Caraway seed	1 tsp.	0.0	.2	0
Cardamom, ground	1 tsp.	0.0	0.0	0
Celery seed	1 tsp.	0.0	.1	0
Chervil, dried	1 tsp.	0.0	0.0	0
Chili powder	1 tsp.	0.0	.3	0
Chives, freeze-dried	1 tsp.	0.0	0.0	0
Cinnamon, ground	1 tsp.	0.0	.4	0
Cloves, ground	1 tsp.	.1	.2	0
Coriander leaf, dried	1 tsp.	0.0	0.0	0
Coriander seed	1 tsp.	0.0	0.0	0
Cumin seed	1 tsp.	0.0	.1	0
Curry powder	1 tsp.	0.0	.2	0
Dill seed	1 tsp.	0.0	.1	0
Dill weed, dried	1 tsp.	0.0	0.0	0
Dill weed, fresh	5 sprigs	0.0	0.0	0
Fennel seed	1 tsp.	0.0	0.0	0
Fenugreek seed	1 tsp.	0.0	0.0	0
Garlic powder	1 tsp.	0.0	0.0	0
Ginger, ground	1 tsp.	0.0	.1	0
Mace, ground	1 tsp.	.2	.1	0
Marjoram, dried	1 tsp.	0.0	0.0	0
Mustard seed, yellow	1 tsp.	0.0	.1	0
Nutmeg, ground	1 tsp.	.6	.1	0
Onion powder	1 tsp.	0.0	0.0	0
Oregano, ground	1 tsp.	0.0	.1	0
Paprika	1 tsp.	0.0	.1	0
Parsley, dried	1 tsp.	0.0	0.0	0
Pepper, black	1 tsp.	0.0	.2	0
Pepper, red cayenne	1 tsp.	.1	.1	0
Pepper, white	1 tsp.	0.0	0.0	0
Poppy seed	1 tsp.	.1	.2	0
Poultry seasoning	1 tsp.	0.0	.1	0
Pumpkin pie spice	1 tsp.	0.0	.1	0

COUNT OUT CHOLESTEROL

Food	Portion	SF1	SF2	Chol
Rosemary, dried	1 tsp.	0.0	0.0	0
Saffron	1 tsp.	0.0	0.0	0
Sage, ground	1 tsp.	0.0	0.0	0
Salt, table	1 tsp.	0.0	0.0	0
Savory, ground	1 tsp.	0.0	0.0	0
Sesame seed, decortic	1 tsp.	0.0	0.0	0
Shallots, freeze-dried	1 tsp.	0.0	0.0	0
Tarragon, ground	1 tsp.	0.0	0.0	0
Thyme, ground	1 tsp.	0.0	.1	0
Tomato powder	1 tsp.	0.0	0.0	0
Turmeric, ground	1 tsp.	0.0	.1	0
Vinegar, cider	1 cup	0.0	0.0	0

SOUPS: CONDENSED OR READY TO USE

Food	Portion	SF1	SF2	Chol
Asparagus, cream of, condensed	8 oz.	2.1	.3	10
Bean/bacon, condensed	8 oz.	3.1	4.8	
Bean, black, condensed	8 oz.	.4	.4	0
Bean/frank, condensed	8 oz.	4.2	3.6	24
Bean/ham, chunky	8 oz.	3.3	3.4	22
Beef broth, ready-to-serve	8 oz.	.3	0.0	0
Beef noodle, condensed	8 oz.	2.3	.5	10
Celery, cream of, condensed	8 oz.	2.8	.5	28
Cheese, condensed	8 oz.	13.3	.6	59
Chicken broth, condensed	8 oz.	.4	0.0	1
Chicken, chunky	8 oz.	2.0	.1	30
Chicken, cream of, condensed, with water	8 oz.	2.0	0.0	10
Chicken, cream of, condensed, with skim milk	8 oz.	4.5	0.0	30
Chicken dumpling, condensed	8 oz.	2.6	0.0	66
Chicken gumbo, condensed	8 oz.	.7	1.2	8
Chicken noodle, chunky	8 oz.	1.4	1.2	19
Chicken noodle, condensed	8 oz.	1.5	.1	10

Food	Portion	SF1	SF2	Chol
Chicken noodle, with meatball, ready-to-serve	8 oz.	1.1	0.0	10
Chicken with rice, chunky	8 oz.	1.0	.3	12
Chicken with rice, condensed	8 oz.	.9	.4	12
Chicken vegetable, chunky	8 oz.	1.4	0.0	17
Chicken vegetable, condensed	8 oz.	1.7	.5	17
Chili/beef, condensed	8 oz.	6.6	0.0	26
Clam chowder, chunky, Manhattan	8 oz.	2.0	.4	10
Clam chowder, condensed, Manhattan	8 oz.	.8	.9	10
Clam chowder, condensed, with skim milk, New England	8 oz.	3.0	.4	20
Consommé, with gel, condensed	8 oz.	0.0	0.0	0
Crab, ready-to-serve	8 oz.	.4	.2	10
Escarole, ready-to-serve	8 oz.	.5	0.0	2
Gazpacho, ready-to-serve	8 oz.	.3	0.5	0
Lentil/ham, ready-to-serve	8 oz.	1.1	0.0	7
Minestrone, chunky, ready-to-serve	8 oz.	1.5	1.0	5
Minestrone, condensed	8 oz.	1.1	.6	2
Mushroom/barley, condensed	8 oz.	.9	0.0	0
Mushroom/beef stock, condensed	8 oz.	3.1	.1	15
Mushroom, cream of, condensed, with water	8 oz.	2.5	.2	2
Mushroom, cream of, condensed, with skim milk	8 oz.	5.0	.2	20
Onion, condensed	8 oz.	.3	.5	0
Onion, cream of, condensed	8 oz.	2.9	.3	30
Oyster stew, condensed	8 oz.	5.0	0.0	27
Pea, green, condensed	8 oz.	2.8	1.5	0
Pea, split & ham, ready-to-serve	8 oz.	1.5	1.5	10

COUNT OUT CHOLESTEROL

Food	Portion	SF1	SF2	Chol
Pea, split & ham, condensed	8 oz.	3.5	1.4	10
Potato, cream of, condensed	8 oz.	2.4	.3	13
Shrimp, cream of, condensed	8 oz.	6.5	.2	33
Stockpot, condensed	8 oz.	1.7	0.0	8
Tomato, condensed, with water	8 oz.	.4	.3	0
Tomato, condensed, with skim milk	8 oz.	3.0	.3	20
Tomato/beef noodle, condensed	8 oz.	3.2	0.0	8
Tomato/rice, condensed	8 oz.	1.0	1.0	3
Turkey, chunky	8 oz.	1.2	0.0	9
Turkey noodle, condensed	8 oz.	1.1	.5	10
Turkey vegetable, condensed	8 oz.	1.8	.4	2
Vegetable, chunky, ready-to-serve	8 oz.	.6	1.5	0
Vegetable, beef, chunky, ready-to-serve	8 oz.	2.5	.4	14
Vegetable, beef, condensed	8 oz.	1.7	1.2	10
Vegetable, beef, broth, condensed	8 oz.	.9	1.0	2
Vegetable, vegetarian, condensed	8 oz.	.5	1.5	0

SOUPS: DEHYDRATED

Food	Portion	SF1	SF2	Chol
Asparagus	8 oz.	.2	.1	0
Bean/bacon	8 oz.	1.0	2.6	3
Bouillon	8 oz.	.3	0.0	1
Bouillon, chicken, cube	8 oz.	.3	0.0	1
Beef broth, cube	8 oz.	.1	0.0	0
Beef noodle	8 oz.	.3	.1	2
Cauliflower	8 oz.	.3	0.0	0
Celery, cream of	8 oz.	.2	.1	1

Food	Portion	SF1	SF2	Chol
Chicken, cream of	8 oz.	3.4	.1	3
Chicken/rice	8 oz.	.3	.1	3
Chicken/vegetable	8 oz.	.2	.1	3
Clam chowder, Manhattan	8 oz.	.3	0.0	0
Clam chowder, New England	8 oz.	.6	.4	1
Consommé, with gel	8 oz.	0.0	0.0	0
Leek	8 oz.	.9	.2	2
Minestrone	8 oz.	.6	.2	1
Oxtail	8 oz.	1.1	0.0	2
Tomato	8 oz.	.9	.1	1
Tomato/vegetable	8 oz.	.4	.2	1
Vegetable/beef	8 oz.	.6	.1	1
Vegetable, cream of	8 oz.	1.4	.2	0

CAKES

Food	Portion	SF1	SF2	Chol
Cakes				
Angel food	1 oz. (1/12 cake)	0.0	.1	0
Angel food, dry mix, prepared	1/12 cake	0.0	0.0	0
Boston cream pie	1/6 of 19.5 oz. pie	2.3	.4	34
Carrot, dry mix, no frosting	1/12 of 9" cake	1.8	0.0	51
Carrot, cream cheese frosting	1/12 of 9" cake	5.4	0.0	60
Cheesecake	1/6 of 17 oz. cake	9.2	.5	44
Cheesecake, mix, no-bake	1/8 of 9" cake	7.0	.6	42
Chocolate, chocolate frosting	1/8 of 18 oz. cake	3.0	.5	29
Chocolate, pudding, dry mix, prepared	1/12 of 9" cake	3.0	0.0	53
Chocolate, regular, dry mix, prepared	1/12 of 9" cake	1.7	0.0	35
Coffeecake, cheese	1/6 of 16 oz. cake	3.8	.3	26
Coffeecake, cinnamon crumb	1/9 of 20 oz. cake	3.6	.6	20

COUNT OUT CHOLESTEROL

Food	Portion	SF1	SF2	Chol
Coffeecake, creme, with chocolate frosting	⅙ of 19 oz. cake	2.5	.5	23
Coffeecake, with fruit	⅛ of 14 oz. cake	1.2	.4	11
Creme-filled, chocolate frosting	1 cupcake	1.6	0.0	9
Fruitcake	1 piece	.5	.5	2
German chocolate, dry mix, frosted	1/12 of 9" cake	5.3	0.0	53
Gingerbread	⅑ of 8" cake	1.0	.5	1
Marble, dry mix, prepared	1/12 of 9" cake	2.3	0.0	53
Pineapple upside-down	⅑ of 8" square cake	3.4	0.0	25
Pound	1 oz. (1/12 cake)	1.3	.1	16
Pound, butter	1 oz. (1/12 cake)	3.2	0.0	63
Shortcake, biscuit	1 shortcake	2.5	0.0	2
Sponge	1/12 of 16 oz. cake	.3	0.0	39
White, pudding, dry mix, prepared	1/12 of 9" cake	1.9	0.0	0
White, regular, dry mix, prepared	1/12 of 9" cake	.7	0.0	0
White, with frosting	1/12 of 9" cake	4.4	0.0	1
Yellow, with chocolate frosting	⅛ of 18 oz. cake	3.0	.3	35
Yellow, with vanilla frosting	⅛ of 18 oz. cake	1.5	0.0	36
Yellow, pudding, dry mix, prepared	1/12 of 9" cake	2.3	0.0	53
Yellow, regular, dry mix, prepared	1/12 of 9" cake	1.0	0.0	37
Frosting				
Chocolate, creamy, ready-to-eat	1/12 package	2.1	0.0	0
Chocolate, creamy, with butter	1/12 package	2.4	0.0	10
Chocolate, creamy, with margarine	1/12 package	.7	0.0	0
Coconut, ready-to-eat	1/12 package	2.7	0.0	0
Cream cheese, ready-to-eat	1/12 package	1.9	0.0	0
Glaze, recipe	1/12 recipe	.5	0.0	1
7-minute, recipe	1/12 recipe	0.0	0.0	0
Sour cream, ready-to-eat	1/12 package	1.9	0.0	0

Food	Portion	SF1	SF2	Chol
Vanilla, creamy, ready-to-eat	¹/₁₂ package	1.9	0.0	0
Vanilla, creamy, with butter	¹/₁₂ package	3.1	0.0	10
Vanilla, creamy, with margarine	¹/₁₂ package	1.4	0.0	0
White, with water	¹/₁₂ package	0.0	0.0	0

COOKIES

Food	Portion	SF1	SF2	Chol
Animal crackers	1 cracker	.1	0.0	0
Brownies	1 brownie	1.5	.3	10
Brownies, dry mix, regular, prepared	1 brownie	1.3	0.0	9
Butter	1 cookie	.5	0.0	4
Cake, fudge	1 cookie	.2	0.0	0
Chocolate wafers	1 wafer	.2	0.0	0
Chocolate chip, lower fat	1 cookie	.4	0.0	0
Chocolate chip, higher fat	1 cookie	.8	.1	0
Chocolate chip, soft	1 cookie	1.1	.1	0
Chocolate chip, dry mix, prepared	2" cookie	1.3	0.0	7
Chocolate chip, refrigerator dough, baked	1 cookie	.9	0.0	3
Chocolate sandwich, creme	1 cookie	.4	.1	0
Chocolate sandwich, extra creme	1 cookie	.6	0.0	0
Coconut macaroon	1 cookie	2.7	0.0	0
Fig Bars	1 cookie	.2	.2	0
Fortune	1 cookie	.1	0.0	1
Ginger snaps	1 cookie	.1	0.0	0
Graham crackers	2.5" square cracker	.5	.5	0
Ladyfingers	1 ladyfinger	.3	0.0	40
Marshmallow	1 small cookie	.6	0.0	0
Molasses	1 medium cookie	.3	0.0	0
Oatmeal	1 cookie	.6	.3	0

Food	Portion	SF1	SF2	Chol
Oatmeal, soft	1 cookie	.4	.1	1
Oatmeal, dry mix, prepared	2" cookie	.8	0.0	7
Oatmeal, refrigerator dough, baked	1 cookie	.6	0.0	3
Peanut butter	1 cookie	.8	0.0	0
Peanut butter, soft	1 cookie	.8	.1	0
Peanut butter, refrigerator dough, baked	1 cookie	.7	0.0	4
Raisin, soft	1 cookie	.5	0.0	0
Shortbread, plain	1 cookie	.5	0.0	2
Shortbread, pecan	1 cookie	1.0	.1	5
Sugar	1 cookie	.8	0.0	8
Sugar, refrigerator dough, baked	1 cookie	.7	0.0	4
Sugar wafers, with creme	1 small wafer	.2	0.0	0
Vanilla sandwich, with creme	1 cookie	.4	0.0	0
Vanilla wafers, lower fat	1 wafer	.1	0.0	2
Vanilla wafers, higher fat	1 wafer	.3	0.0	0
Pastries				
Cream puff, shell	1 shell	3.7	0.0	129
Cream puff, with custard	1 cream puff	4.8	0.0	174
Danish, cinnamon	1 pastry	3.7	.2	20
Danish, cheese	1 pastry	4.9	0.0	32
Danish, fruit	1 pastry	3.3	.4	15
Danish, nut	1 pastry	3.5	.4	30
Donut, cake, plain	1 medium	2.4	.2	20
Donut, cake, chocolate, frosted	1 medium	3.6	.3	25
Donut, cake, chocolate, sugar/glazed	1 medium	2.3	.3	24
Donut, cake, white, sugar/glazed	1 medium	1.4	0.0	9
Donut, French cruller, glazed	1 cruller	1.9	0.0	5
Donut, yeast-leavened, cream	1 donut	5.7	0.0	20

Food	Portion	SF1	SF2	Chol
Donut, yeast-leavened, glazed	1 medium	3.5	.4	4
Donut, yeast-leavened, jelly	1 donut	4.0	0.0	22
Eclairs	1 eclair	4.1	0.0	127
Hushpuppies	1 hushpuppy	.5	.2	10
Ice cream cone, sugar	1 cone	.1	.1	0
Ice cream cone, wafer	1 cone	0.0	0.0	0

PIES

Food	Portion	SF1	SF2	Chol
Apple	1/8 of 9" pie	3.4	1.5	0
Banana creme, mix, no-bake	1/8 of 9" pie	6.4	0.0	25
Blueberry	1/8 of 9" pie	2.3	0.0	0
Cherry	1/8 of 9" pie	2.6	.3	0
Chocolate creme	1/6 of 8" pie	6.0	.7	6
Chocolate mousse, mix, no-bake	1/8 of 9" pie	7.8	0.0	21
Coconut creme	1/6 of 7" pie	4.8	0.0	0
Coconut creme, mix, no-bake	1/8 of 9" pie	9.6	0.0	24
Coconut custard	1/6 of 8" pie	6.0	.6	36
Egg custard	1/6 of 8" pie	2.9	.4	35
Fried pies, fruit	1 pie	3.1	1.0	0
Lemon meringue	1/6 of 9" pie	4.5	.5	140
Mince	1/8 of 9" pie	4.4	0.0	0
Peach	1/6 of 8" pie	2.2	0.0	0
Pecan	1/6 of 8" pie	4.2	1.2	36
Pumpkin	1/6 of 8" pie	2.2	.9	22
Vanilla creme	1/8 of 9" pie	5.1	0.0	78
Pie crust, chocolate wafer, baked	1/8 of 9" crust	1.9	0.0	1
Pie crust, graham cracker, baked	1/8 of 9" crust	1.6	0.0	0
Pie crust, vanilla wafer, baked	1/8 of 9" crust	1.7	0.0	9
Pie crust, dry mix, baked	1/8 of 9" crust	1.5	0.0	0

Food	Portion	SF1	SF2	Chol
Pie crust, frozen, ready-to-bake, baked	⅛ of 9" crust	1.7	0.0	0
Phyllodough	1 sheet	.2	0.0	0
Popovers, dry mix, prepared	1 popover	.4	0.0	37
Popovers, 2% milk	1 popover	.8	0.0	46
Strudel, apple	1 strudel	2.1	.5	20
Sweet roll, cheese	1 roll	3.8	0.0	37
Sweet roll, cinnamon/raisin	1 roll	2.5	.2	40
Sweet roll, cinnamon, refrigerator dough, baked, frosted	1 roll	1.0	0.0	0
Sweet roll, raisin+nuts	1 roll	1.4	0.0	13
Toaster pastry, brown sugar/cinnamon	1 pastry	1.8	0.0	0
Toaster pastry, fruit	1 pastry	.8	0.0	0

SNACKS

Food	Portion	SF1	SF2	Chol
Banana Chips	1 oz.	8.2	.7	0
Beef jerky	1 oz.	1.7	0.0	32
Chex mix	⅔ cup (1 oz.)	0.0	0.0	0
Corn chips, plain	1 oz.	1.5	.1	0
Corn chips, bbq	1 oz.	1.3	.4	0
Corn cones, plain	1 oz.	6.4	0.0	0
Corn cones, nacho	1 oz.	7.6	0.0	1
Corn snacks, onion	1 oz.	1.2	.3	0
Corn puffs, cheese	1 oz.	1.9	.1	1
Cornnuts, plain	1 oz.	.7	.6	0
Cornnuts, bbq	1 oz.	.7	.7	0
Cornnuts, nacho	1 oz.	.7	.7	1
Doo Dads, original flavor	½ cup (1 oz.)	0.0	.6	0
Fried pie, fruit	1 pie	6.5	0.0	13
Fruit leather, bars	1 bar	.9	0.0	0
Fruit leather, bars, with cream	1 bar	.6	0.0	1
Fruit leather, pieces	1 oz.	.3	0.0	0

Food	Portion	SF1	SF2	Chol
Fruit leather, rolls	1 small roll	.1	0.0	0
Granola bar, hard, plain	1 bar	.7	.5	0
Granola bar, hard, almond	1 bar	3.0	0.0	0
Granola bar, hard, chocolate chip	1 bar	2.7	.3	0
Granola bar, hard, peanut	1 bar	.6	0.0	0
Granola bar, soft, plain	1 bar	2.1	.4	0
Granola bar, soft, chocolate chip	1 bar	4.0	.3	1
Granola bar, soft, peanut	1 bar	1.0	.4	0
Granola bar, soft, peanut butter	1 bar	6.2	0.0	4
Granola bar, soft, raisin	1 bar	2.7	.4	0
Meat-based sticks, smoked	1 oz.	5.9	0.0	38
Oriental mix, rice-based	1 oz.	5.0	1.1	0
Popcorn, air-popped	1 cup	0.0	.3	0
Popcorn, oil-popped	1 cup	.5	.3	0
Popcorn, cakes	1 cake	0.0	.1	0
Popcorn, caramel-coated, with peanuts	1 oz. (⅔ cup)	.3	.3	0
Popcorn, caramel-coated, no peanuts	1 cup	1.3	.5	2
Popcorn, cheese	1 cup	.7	.3	1
Pork skins, plain	1 oz.	3.2	0.0	27
Pork skins, bbq	1 oz.	3.3	0.0	33
Potato chip	1 oz.	2.5	.1	0
Potato chip, bbq	1 oz.	2.3	.4	0
Potato chip, light	1 oz.	1.5	.3	0
Potato chip, sour cream & onion	1 oz.	2.5	.4	2
Pretzels, combos, cheddar	1 oz.	0.0	0.0	3
Pretzels, hard, plain, salted	1 oz.	.2	.3	0
Pretzels, hard, chocolate coating	1 oz.	2.2	0.0	0
Pretzels, hard, whole-wheat	1 oz.	.2	0.0	0
Rice cake, brown rice, plain	1 cake	.1	.1	0
Rice cake, brown rice, buckwheat	1 cake	.1	.1	0

COUNT OUT CHOLESTEROL

Food	Portion	SF1	SF2	Chol
Rice cake, brown rice, sesame seed	1 cake	0.0	.1	0
Tortilla chip, plain	1 oz.	1.4	.6	0
Tortilla chip, nacho	1 oz.	1.4	.5	1
Tortilla chip, ranch	1 oz.	1.3	0.0	0
Trail mix, chocolate chip, salted	1 oz.	1.7	0.0	1
Trail mix, regular	1 oz.	1.6	0.0	0
Trail mix, tropical	1 oz.	2.4	0.0	0

CANDY

Food	Portion	SF1	SF2	Chol
After Eight Mints	2 pieces	.7	0.0	0
Almond Joy candy	1 snack size bar	3.3	0.0	0
	1 bar (1.76 oz.)	8.3	0.0	1
Alpine White bar with almonds	1 bar (1.25 oz.)	6.7	.6	4
Baby Ruth	1 bar (2.1 oz.)	6.9	.5	14
Baking chocolate, unsweetened, square	1 oz.	9.5	.2	0
Bar None	1 bar (1.5 oz.)	0.0	.4	7
Bit-o-Honey Chews	1 bar (1.7 oz.)	0.0	0.0	0
Butterfinger	1 snack size bar	1.8	.2	0
	1 bar (2.16 oz.)	5.2	.5	1
Butterscotch	1 piece	.1	0.0	1
Caramello	1 bar (1.6 oz.)	0.0	0.0	11
	1 bar (5 oz.)	0.0	0.0	34
Caramels	1 piece	.5	0.0	1
Caramels, chocolate, roll	1 piece	0.0	0.0	0
Carob	1 oz.	2.4	.5	1
Chewing gum	1 stick	0.0	0.0	0
Chunky	1 bar (1.25 oz.)	8.1	.5	4
Demet's Turtles	1 piece	1.8	0.0	4
5th Avenue	1 bar (2.1 oz.)	0.0	0.0	2
Fudge, chocolate	1 oz.	2.0	0.0	1
Golden Almond	1 bar (3 oz.)	0.0	0.0	10
Golden Almond Solitaires	1 package (3 oz.)	0.0	0.0	10

Food	Portion	SF1	SF2	Chol
Golden III chocolate bar	1 bar (3.2 oz.)	0.0	0.0	17
Goobers Chocolate-covered				
Peanuts	1 package (1.38 oz.)	4.8	0.0	4
Gumdrops	10 large	0.0	0.0	0
Hard candy	1 oz.	0.0	0.0	0
Jellybeans	1 oz.	0.0	0.0	0
Kit Kat	1 bar (1.6 oz.)	7.7	.1	12
	1 bar (3.4 oz.)	16.0	.3	24
Krackel	1 bar (1.65 oz.)	5.6	0.0	9
	1 bar (2.6 oz.)	8.7	0.0	14
Mars Almond	1 bar (1.76 oz.)	0.0	.3	5
Marshmallows	1 cup	0.0	0.0	0
Mars Milky Way	1 snack size bar	1.4	.1	4
	1 bar (2.1 oz.)	4.7	.3	12
Milk chocolate,				
with almonds	1 bar (1.45 oz.)	7.0	.8	8
	1 bar (1.55 oz.)	7.5	.8	8
Milk chocolate, with rice	1 bar (1.4 oz.)	6.4	.3	8
	1 bar (1.45 oz.)	7.2	.4	9
"M&M's" Peanut	1 package (1.74 oz.)	0.0	.5	6
"M&M's" Plain	1 package (1.69 oz.)	0.0	.4	7
Mounds	1 snack size bar	2.3	.2	0
	1 package (1.9 oz.)	6.2	.5	0
Mr. Goodbar	1 bar (1.75 oz.)	9.0	.6	10
	1 bar (2.8 oz.)	14.3	1.0	16
Nestle Crunch	1 snack size bar	1.4	.1	2
	1 bar (1.4 oz.)	5.7	.3	8
Oh Henry!	1 bar (2 oz.)	3.8	.6	5
Peanut bar	1 bar (1.4 oz.)	1.7	.4	3
	1 bar (1.6 oz.)	1.9	.4	3
Peanut brittle	1 oz.	1.4	.2	4
Raisinets	1 package (1.58 oz.)	3.3	0.0	2
Reese's Peanut Buttercups	1 package (1.8 oz.)	11.8	.6	8
Reese's Pieces	1 package (1.95 oz.)	0.0	.7	2
Rolo Caramels	1 package (1.93 oz.)	0.0	.1	13
Sesame Crunch	1 oz.	1.3	.7	0
Skittles	1 package (2.3 oz.)	0.0	0.0	0
Skor Toffee Candy	1 bar (1.4 oz.)	0.0	0.0	24
Snickers	1 snack size bar	1.8	.1	2
	1 bar (2.16 oz.)	7.3	.5	7

COUNT OUT CHOLESTEROL

Food	Portion	SF1	SF2	Chol
Special Dark				
Sweet Chocolate	1 bar (1.45 oz.)	0.0	.7	0
	1 bar (2.8 oz.)	0.0	1.3	0
Starburst Fruit Chews	1 package (2.07 oz.)	0.0	0.0	0
Symphony Milk Chocolate	1 bar (1.4 oz.)	0.0	0.0	11
	1 bar (2.4 oz.)	0.0	0.0	19
3 Musketeers	1 snack size bar	1.2	.1	2
	1 bar (2.13 oz.)	3.9	.3	7
Truffles, recipe	1 piece	2.6	0.0	6
	1 bar (1.4 oz.)	5.7	.3	8
Twix Caramel	1 package (2 oz.)	0.0	.3	5
Twix Peanut Butter	1 package (1.77 oz.)	0.0	.5	6
Whatchamacallit	1 bar (1.8 oz.)	0.0	.5	11
Y&S Nibs Cherry Candy	1 oz.	0.0	0.0	0
Y&S Twizzlers, strawberry	1 package (2.5 oz.)	0.0	0.0	0
	1 package (5 oz.)	0.0	0.0	0
York Peppermint Patty	1 small patty	0.0	0.0	0
	1 large patty	0.0	0.0	0

CUSTARDS, GELATINS, PUDDINGS

Food	Portion	SF1	SF2	Chol
Egg custard, baked	½ cup	3.0	0.0	123
Flan, caramel custard	½ cup	3.0	0.0	141
Gelatin, dry, with water	½ cup	0.0	0.0	0
Gelatin, dry, with fruit	½ cup	.1	0.0	0
Pudding, banana, 2% milk	½ cup	1.5	0.0	10
Pudding, banana, ready-to-eat	1 can (5 oz.)	.8	0.0	0
Pudding, bread, recipe	½ cup	2.9	0.0	83
Pudding, chocolate, with whole milk	½ cup	2.7	.4	16
Pudding, chocolate, 2% milk	½ cup	2.0	0.0	9
Pudding, chocolate, ready-to-eat	1 container (5 oz.)	1.0	.4	4
Pudding, coconut, instant, with whole milk	½ cup	3.1	0.0	16

Food	Portion	SF1	SF2	Chol
Pudding, coconut cream, instant, with 2% milk	½ cup	2.0	0.0	9
Pudding, lemon, instant, with whole milk	½ cup	2.6	0.0	16
Pudding, lemon, instant, 2% milk	½ cup	1.5	0.0	9
Pudding, rice, mix, with whole milk	½ cup	2.5	0.0	16
Pudding, rice, ready-to-eat	1 can (5 oz.)	1.7	0.0	1
Pudding, tapioca	½ cup	2.5	0.0	20
Pudding, tapioca, ready-to-eat	1 container (5 oz.)	.9	0.0	1
Pudding, vanilla, instant, with whole milk	½ cup	2.5	0.0	16
Pudding, vanilla, instant, with 2% milk	½ cup	1.4	0.0	9
Pudding, vanilla, ready-to-eat	½ cup	.6	0.0	8

ICE CREAM AND FROZEN DESSERTS

Food	Portion	SF1	SF2	Chol
Frozen fruit & juice bars	1 bar (3 oz.)	0.0	0.0	0
Frozen pudding pops, chocolate	1 pop	0.0	.1	1
Frozen pudding pops, vanilla	1 pop	0.0	0.0	1
Ice cream, chocolate	½ cup	4.5	0.0	22
Ice cream, strawberry	½ cup	0.0	0.0	19
Ice cream, vanilla	½ cup	4.5	0.0	30
Ice cream, vanila, rich	½ cup	7.4	0.0	45
Ice milk, vanilla, soft serve	½ cup	1.4	0.0	11
Ice milk, vanilla	½ cup	1.7	0.0	9
Ices, fruit	½ cup	0.0	0.0	0
Ice Pops	1 bar (2 oz.)	0.0	0.0	0
Sherbet, orange	½ cup	1.2	.1	5
Sundae, caramel	1 sundae	4.5	0.0	25
Sundae, hot fudge	1 sundae	5.0	0.0	21

Food	Portion	SF1	SF2	Chol
Sundae, strawberry	1 sundae	3.7	0.0	21
Yogurt, frozen, chocolate, soft serve	½ cup	2.6	0.0	4
Yogurt, frozen, vanilla, soft serve	½ cup	2.5	0.0	1

ALCOHOLIC BEVERAGES

Food	Portion	SF1	SF2	Chol
Beer	12 oz.	0.0	.2	0
Wine	5 oz.	0.0	0.0	0
Distilled spirits 80 proof	1 oz.	0.0	0.0	0
Bloody Mary	5 oz.	0.0	0.0	0
Daiquiri	5 oz.	0.0	0.0	0
Gin and Tonic	5 oz.	0.0	0.0	0
Martini	5 oz.	0.0	0.0	0
Piña Colada	5 oz.	1.5	0.0	0
Piña Colada, canned	6.8 oz.	14.6	.1	0
Screwdriver	5 oz.	0.0	0.0	0

NON-ALCOHOLIC BEVERAGES

Food	Portion	SF1	SF2	Chol
Carob flavored beverage with milk	1 cup milk +3 tsp. powder	5.1	0.0	33
Chocolate flavored beverage with milk	1 cup milk +3 tsp. powder	5.5	0.0	32
Chocolate malt & milk	1 cup milk +5 heaping tsp.	5.5	0.0	34
Chocolate syrup & milk	1 cup milk +2 tbsp. syrup	5.3	0.0	34
Citrus drink, frozen, diluted	1 cup	0.0	0.0	0
Club soda	12 oz.	0.0	0.0	0
Cocoa mix & water	6 oz. +4 tsp. powder	.7	.7	2

Food	Portion	SF1	SF2	Chol
Coffee	6 oz.	0.0	0.0	0
Coffee & sugar (cappuccino) powder	2 rounded tsp.	1.8	0.0	0
Coffee & sugar (mocha) powder	2 rounded tsp.	1.6	0.0	0
Colas	12 oz.	0.0	0.0	0
Cranberry cocktail, bottled	1 cup	.1	.1	0
Eggnog mix & milk	1 cup milk +2 heaping tsp.	5.1	0.0	33
Fruit punch, canned	1 cup	0.0	0.0	0
Fruit punch, frozen, prepared	1 cup	0.0	0.0	0
Fruit punch, powder & water	1 cup water +2 tsp. powder	0.0	0.0	0
Gelatin powder, orange	1 packet	0.0	0.0	0
Grape drink, canned	1 cup	0.0	0.0	0
Grape juice drink, canned	1 cup	0.0	.1	0
Lemonade, frozen, diluted	1 cup	0.0	0.0	0
Lemonade, powder+water	1 cup water+2 tbsp.	0.0	0.0	0
Limeade, frozen, prepared	1 cup	0.0	0.0	0
Malt beverage	1 cup	0.0	0.0	0
Milk shake, chocolate (fastfood)	10 oz.	6.5	0.2	40
Milk shake, strawberry (fastfood)	10 oz.	4.9	0.0	31
Milk shake, vanilla (fastfood)	10 oz.	5.3	0.0	31
Natural malt & milk	1 cup milk +5 heaping tsp.	5.4	0.0	34
Orange breakfast drink, frozen, prepared	1 cup	0.0	0.0	0
Orange drink, canned	1 cup	0.0	.1	0
Orange drink, frozen, prepared	1 cup	0.0	0.0	0
Sodas	12 oz.	0.0	0.0	0
Strawberry mix & milk	1 cup milk +3 heaping tsp.	5.1	0.0	32
Tea, brewed	6 oz.	0.0	0.0	0
Tonic water	12 oz.	0.0	0.0	0

MISCELLANEOUS

Food	Portion	SF1	SF2	Chol
Cocoa, dry powder, unsweetened	1 tbsp.	.5	.2	0
Fruit butter, apple	1 tbsp.	0.0	.1	0
Honey	1 tbsp.	0.0	0.0	0
Jams & preserves	1 tbsp.	0.0	.1	0
Jellies	1 tbsp.	0.0	.1	0
Marmalade, orange	1 tbsp.	0.0	0.0	0
Molasses	1 tbsp.	0.0	0.0	0
Pectin, unsweetened, mix	1 package (1.75 oz.)	0.0	0.0	0
Sugar, brown	1 cup	0.0	0.0	0
Sugar, granulated	1 cup	0.0	0.0	0
Sugar, powdered	1 cup	0.0	0.0	0
Syrups, chocolate, fudge	1 tbsp.	1.2	.1	3
Syrups, corn	1 cup	0.0	0.0	0
Syrups, maple	1 tbsp.	0.0	0.0	0
Syrups, pancake	1 tbsp.	0.0	0.0	0
Syrups, pancake, with butter	1 tbsp.	.2	0.0	1
Syrups, pancake, reduced calorie	1 tbsp.	0.0	0.0	0
Topping, butterscotch/caramel	2 tbsp.	0.0	0.0	0
Topping, marshmallow creme	2 tbsp.	0.0	0.0	0
Topping, pineapple	2 tbsp.	0.0	.1	0
Topping, strawberry	2 tbsp.	0.0	0.0	0

FAST FOODS
(Common breakfast and lunch menu items)

Food	Portion	SF1	SF2	Chol
Biscuit, with egg	1 biscuit	6.2	0.0	233
Biscuit, with egg+bacon	1 biscuit	9.9	0.0	353
Biscuit, with egg, bacon+cheese	1 biscuit	11.4	0.0	261
Biscuit, with egg+ham	1 biscuit	8.4	0.0	300
Biscuit, with egg+sausage	1 biscuit	15.0	0.0	302

Food	Portion	SF1	SF2	Chol
Biscuit, with ham	1 biscuit	11.4	0.0	25
Biscuit, with sausage	1 biscuit	14.2	.4	35
Biscuit, with steak	1 biscuit	6.9	0.0	25
Burrito, with beans	2 burritos	6.9	0.0	4
Burrito, with beans+cheese	2 burritos	6.8	0.0	28
Burrito, with beans, cheese+peppers	2 burritos	11.2	0.0	158
Burrito, with beans+peppers	2 burritos	7.6	0.0	33
Burrito, with beans, beef+cheese	2 burritos	7.1	0.0	124
Burrito, with beef	2 burritos	10.5	0.0	64
Burrito, with beef, cheese+peppers	2 burritos	10.4	0.0	170
Burrito, with beef+peppers	2 burritos	8.0	0.0	54
Cheeseburger, regular, single, plain	1 burger	6.5	0.0	50
Cheeseburger, with condiments	1 burger	6.3	0.0	37
Cheeseburger, with condiments+vegetables	1 burger	9.2	0.0	52
Cheeseburger, double meat	1 burger	13.0	0.0	110
Cheeseburger, double meat, with condiments+vegetables	1 burger	8.7	0.0	60
Cheeseburger, double meat, double bun	1 burger	9.5	0.0	80
Cheeseburger, double meat, with condiments+vegetables	1 burger	12.8	0.0	93
Cheeseburger, large, plain	1 burger	14.8	0.0	96
Cheeseburger, large, with bacon+condiments	1 burger	16.2	0.0	111
Cheeseburger, large, with condiments+vegetables	1 burger	15.0	0.0	88
Cheeseburger, large, double meat, with vegetables	1 burger	17.7	0.0	142
Cheeseburger, large, triple meat, plain	1 burger	21.7	0.0	161

Food	Portion	SF1	SF2	Chol
Chicken fillet sandwich, plain	1 sandwich	8.5	0.0	60
Chicken fillet sandwich, with cheese	1 sandwich	12.4	0.0	78
Chicken, fried, dark meat	2 pieces	7.0	0.0	166
Chicken, fried, light meat	2 pieces	7.8	0.0	148
Chicken, fried, no bone	6 pieces	5.5	.1	61
Chicken piece, with bbq sauce	6 pieces	5.6	0.0	61
Chicken piece, with honey	6 pieces	5.5	0.0	61
Chicken piece, with mustard sauce	6 pieces	5.7	0.0	61
Chicken piece, with sweet+sour sauce	6 pieces	5.5	0.0	61
Chili Con Carne	8 oz. cup	3.4	0.0	134
Chimichanga, with beef	1 chimichanga	8.5	0.0	9
Chimichanga, with beef+cheese	1 chimichanga	11.2	0.0	51
Chimichanga, with beef, cheese+peppers	1 chimichanga	8.4	0.0	50
Chimichanga, with beef+peppers	1 chimichanga	8.3	0.0	10
Coleslaw	¾ cup	1.6	0.0	5
Corn dog	1 hot dog	5.2	0.0	79
Corn-on-the-cob, with butter	1 ear	1.6	0.0	6
Croissant, with egg+cheese	1 croissant	14.1	0.0	216
Croissant, with egg, cheese+bacon	1 croissant	15.4	0.0	215
Croissant, with egg, cheese+ham	1 croissant	17.5	0.0	213
Croissant, with egg, cheese+sausage	1 croissant	18.2	0.0	216
Egg+cheese sandwich	1 sandwich	6.6	0.0	291
Egg, scrambled	2 eggs	5.8	0.0	400
Enchilada, cheese	1 enchilada	10.6	0.0	44
Enchilada, cheese+beef	1 enchilada	9.0	0.0	40
Enchirito, cheese, beef+beans	1 enchirito	7.9	0.0	50

Food	Portion	SF1	SF2	Chol
English muffin, with cheese+sausage	1 muffin	9.9	0.0	59
English muffin, with egg, cheese+bacon	1 muffin	9.1	0.0	234
English muffin, with egg, cheese+sausage	1 muffin	12.4	0.0	274
Fish sandwich, with tartar sauce	1 sandwich	5.2	0.0	55
Fish sandwich, with tartar sauce+cheese	1 sandwich	8.1	0.0	68
Frijoles, with cheese	8 oz. cup	4.1	0.0	37
Ham+cheese sandwich	1 sandwich	6.4	0.0	58
Ham, cheese+egg sandwich	1 sandwich	7.4	0.0	246
Hamburger, regular, plain	1 burger	4.1	0.0	35
Hamburger, regular, with condiments	1 burger	3.5	0.0	43
Hamburger, regular, with condiments+vegetables	1 burger	4.1	0.0	26
Hamburger, double meat	1 burger	10.4	0.0	99
Hamburger, double meat, with condiments	1 burger	12.0	0.0	103
Hamburger, large, single, plain	1 burger	8.4	0.0	71
Hamburger, large, double meat, with vegetables	1 burger	10.5	0.0	122
Hamburger, large, triple meat, with condiments	1 burger	15.9	0.0	142
Hot dog, plain	1 hot dog	5.1	0.0	44
Hot dog, with chili	1 hot dog	4.9	0.0	51
Hushpuppies	5 hushpuppies	2.7	0.0	135
Nachos, with cheese	6-8 nachos	7.8	0.0	18
Nachos, with cheese+peppers	6-8 nachos	14.0	0.0	84
Nachos, with cheese, beans, beef+peppers	6-8 nachos	12.5	0.0	20

COUNT OUT CHOLESTEROL

Food	Portion	SF1	SF2	Chol
Nachos,				
with cinnamon+sugar	6-8 nachos	18.2	0.0	39
Onion rings, fried	8-9 onion rings	7.0	0.0	14
Pizza, with cheese	1 slice	1.5	0.0	20
Pizza, with cheese,				
meat+vegetables	1 slice	1.5	0.0	35
Pizza, with pepperoni	1 slice	2.2	0.0	32
Potato, baked,				
with cheese sauce	1 potato	10.6	0.0	18
Potato, baked,				
with cheese+bacon	1 potato	10.1	0.0	30
Potato, baked,				
with cheese+broccoli	1 potato	8.5	0.0	20
Potato, baked,				
with cheese+chili	1 potato	13.0	0.0	32
Potato, baked,				
with sour cream+chives	1 potato	10.0	0.0	24
Potato, fried				
with animal fat	regular order	5.6	0.0	14
Potato, fried with animal				
+vegetable fat	regular order	5.0	0.0	11
	large order	7.6	0.0	16
Potato, fried				
with vegetable oil	regular order	3.8	0.0	0
	large order	5.7	0.0	0
Potatoes, hash brown	½ cup	4.3	0.0	9
Potato, mashed	⅓ cup	.4	0.0	2
Potato salad	⅓ cup	1.0	0.0	57
Roast beef sandwich	1 sandwich	3.6	0.0	51
Roast beef sandwich,				
with cheese	1 sandwich	9.0	0.0	77
Salad, vegetable, no dressing	1½ cups	0.0	0.0	0
Salad, with cheese+egg	1½ cups	3.0	0.0	98
Salad, with chicken	1½ cups	.6	0.0	72
Salad, with pasta+seafood	1½ cups	2.6	0.0	50
Salad, with shrimp	1½ cups	.7	0.0	179

Food	Portion	SF1	SF2	Chol
Salad, with turkey, ham+cheese	1½ cups	8.2	0.0	140
Steak sandwich	1 sandwich	1.9	0.0	36
Sub, cold cut	1 sub	6.8	0.0	36
Sub, roast beef	1 sub	7.1	0.0	73
Sub, tuna salad	1 sub	5.3	0.0	49
Taco	1 small	11.4	0.0	56
	1 large	17.5	0.0	87
Taco salad	1½ cups	6.8	0.0	44
Taco salad, with chili	1½ cups	6.0	0.0	5
Tostada, with beans+cheese	1 tostada	5.4	0.0	30
Tostada, with beans, cheese+beef	1 tostada	11.5	0.0	74
Tostada, with beef+cheese	1 tostada	10.4	0.0	41
Tostada, with guacamole	2 tostadas	9.9	0.0	39

♥ ♥ ♥ ♥

REFERENCES

Chapter 1

Ernst, Nancy D. "NIH Consensus Development Conference on Lowering Blood Cholesterol to Prevent Heart Disease: Implications for Dietitians." *Journal of the American Dietetic Association* 85 (1985): 586-88.

Marniemi, Jukka, et al. "Metabolic Changes Induced by Combined Prolonged Exercise and Low-Calorie Intake in Man." *European Journal of Applied Physiology* 53 (1984): 121-27.

National Cholesterol Education Program. *Report of the Expert Panel on Detection, Evaluation, and Treatment of High Blood Cholesterol in Adults.* NIH Publication No. 88-2925, 1988.

National Heart, Lung, and Blood Institute Consensus Development Panel (NIH). "Lowering Blood Cholesterol to Prevent Heart Disease." *JAMA* 253 (1985): 2080-86.

National Heart, Lung, and Blood Institute, U.S. Department of Health and Human Services. *So You Have High Cholesterol . . . .* NIH Publication No. 87-2922, 1987.

Chapter 2

Blankenhorn, David H., et al. "The Influence of Diet on the Appearance of New Lesions in Human Coronary Arteries." *JAMA* 263 (1990): 1646-52.

Brensike, John F., et al. "Effects of Therapy with Cholestyramine on Progression of Coronary Arteriosclerosis: Results of the NHLBI Type II Coronary Intervention Study." *Circulation* 69 (1984): 313-24.

Castelli, William P., et al. "A Population at Risk." *American Journal of Medicine* 62 (1977): 707-14.

———. "Incidence of Coronary Heart Disease and Lipoprotein Cholesterol Levels—The Framingham Study." *JAMA* 256 (1986): 2835-38.

Expert Panel on Detection, Evaluation, and Treatment of High Blood Cholesterol in Adults. "Summary of the Second Report of the National Cholesterol Education Program (NCEP) Expert Panel on Detection, Evaluation, and Treatment of High Blood Cholesterol in Adults (Adult Treatment Panel II)." *JAMA* 269 (1993): 3015-23.

Frick, M. Heikki, et al. "Helsinki Heart Study: Primary-Prevention Trial Results." *New England Journal of Medicine* 317 (1987): 1237-45.

Gordon, Tavia, et al. "High Density Lipoprotein as a Protective Factor Against Coronary Heart Disease." *American Journal of Medicine* 62 (1977): 707-14.

Keys, Ancel, ed. "Coronary Heart Disease in Seven Countries." *Circulation* 41 (1970): supp. 1, 1-211.

Keys, Ancel, et al. "HDL Serum Cholesterol and 24-Year Mortality of Men in Finland." *International Journal of Epidemiology* 13 (1984): 428-35.

Lipid Research Clinics Program. "The Lipid Research Clinics Coronary Primary Prevention Trial Results: I. Reduction in Incidence of Coronary Heart Disease." *JAMA* 251 (1984): 351-64.

———. "The Lipid Research Clinics Coronary Primary Prevention Results: II. The Relationship of Reduction in Incidence of Coronary Heart Disease to Cholesterol Lowering." *JAMA* 251 (1984): 365-74.

Martin, Michael J., et al. "Serum Cholesterol, Blood Pressure, and Mortality: Implications from a Cohort of 361,662 Men." *Lancet* 2 (1984): 933-36.

Ornish, Dean, et al. "Can Lifestyle Changes Reverse Coronary Heart Disease?" *Lancet* 336 (1990): 129-33.

Stamler, Jeremiah, et al. "Is Relationship Between Serum Cholesterol and Risk of Premature Death from Coronary Heart Disease Continuous and Graded?" *JAMA* 256 (1986): 2823-28.

REFERENCES

Watts, G.F., et al. "Effects on Coronary Artery Disease of Lipid-Lowering Diet, or Diet Plus Cholestyramine, in the St. Thomas' Atherosclerosis Regression Study (STARS)." *Lancet* 339 (1992): 563-69.

Chapter 3

Ahrens, Edward H. "The Influence of Dietary Fats on Serum-Lipid Levels in Man." *Lancet* 1 (1957): 943-53.

American Medical Association Council on Scientific Affairs. "Dietary and Pharmacologic Therapy for the Lipid Risk Factors." *JAMA* 250 (1983): 1873-79.

Anderson, James W., et al. "Fiber and Health: An Overview."*American Journal of Gastroenterology* 81 (1986): 892-97.

———. "Prospective, Randomized, Controlled Comparison of the Effects of Low-Fat and Low-Fat Plus High-Fiber Diets on Serum Lipid Concentrations." *American Journal of Clinical Nutrition* 56 (1992): 887-94.

Barr, Susan, et al. "Reducing Total Dietary Fat without Reducing Saturated Fatty Acids Does Not Significantly Lower Total Plasma Cholesterol Concentrations in Normal Males." *American Journal of Clinical Nutrition* 55 (1992): 675-81.

Brown, W. Virgil, et al. "Treatment of Common Lipoprotein Disorders." *Progress in Cardiovascular Diseases* 27 (1984): 1-20.

Caggiula, Arlene W., et al. "The Multiple Risk Factor Intervention Trial (MRFIT). IV. Intervention on Blood Lipids." *Preventive Medicine* 10 (1981): 443-75.

Ehnholm, Christian, et al. "Effect of Diet on Serum Lipoproteins in a Population with a High Risk of Coronary Heart Disease." *New England Journal of Medicine* 307 (1982): 850-55.

Grundy, Scott, et al. "Comparison of Monounsaturated Fatty Acids and Carbohydrates for Reducing Raised Levels of Plasma Cholesterol in Man." *American Journal of Clinical Nutrition* 47 (1988): 965-69.

———. "Rationale of the Diet-Heart Statement of the American Heart Association: Report of the Nutrition Committee." *Circulation* 65 (1982): 839A-54A.

———. "Trans Monounsaturated Fatty Acids and Serum Cholesterol Levels." *New England Journal of Medicine* 323 (1990): 480-81.

Jenkins, David J.A., et al. "Effect on Blood Lipids of Very High Intakes of Fiber in Diets Low in Saturated Fat and Cholesterol." *New England Journal of Medicine* 329 (1993): 21-26.

Keys, Ancel, et al. "Prediction of Serum-Cholesterol Responses of Man to Changes in Fats in the Diet." *Lancet* 1 (1957): 959-66.

————. "Serum Cholesterol Response to Dietary Fat." *Lancet* 2 (1957): 787.

————. "Serum Cholesterol Response to Changes in the Diet. II: The Effect of Cholesterol in the Diet." *Metabolism* 14 (1965): 759-87.

Khaw, Kay-Tee, et al. "Dietary Fiber and Reduced Ischemic Heart Disease Mortality Rates in Men and Women: A Twelve-Year Prospective Study." *American Journal of Epidemiology* 126 (1987): 1093-1102.

Mattson, Fred H., et al. "Comparison of Effects of Dietary Saturated, Monounsaturated, and Polyunsaturated Fatty Acids on Plasma Lipids and Lipoproteins in Man." *Journal of Lipid Research* 26 (1985): 194-202.

Mensink, R.P., et al. "Effect of Dietary Trans Fatty Acids on High-Density and Low-Density Lipoprotein Cholesterol Levels in Healthy Subjects." *New England Journal of Medicine* 323 (1990): 439-45.

Multiple Risk Factor Intervention Trial Research Group. "Multiple Risk Factor Intervention Trial: Risk Factor Changes and Mortality Results." *JAMA* 248 (1982): 1465-77.

Schaefer, Ernst J., et al. "The Effects of Low Cholesterol, High Polyunsaturated Fat, and Low Fat Diets on Plasma Lipid and Lipoprotein Cholesterol Levels in Normal and Hypercholesterolemic Subjects." *American Journal of Clinical Nutrition* 34 (1981): 1758-63.

————. "Prediction of Serum-Cholesterol Responses of Man to Changes in Fats in the Diet." *Lancet* (1957): 959-66.

Chapter 4

Schucker, Beth. "Change in Physician Perspective on Cholesterol and Heart Disease: Results from Two National Surveys." *JAMA* 258 (1987): 3527-31.

Wilson, Peter W.F. "Coronary Risk Prediction in Adults (The Framingham Heart Study)." *American Journal of Cardiology* 59 (1987): 91G-94G.

Chapter 6

Oxley, Dwight K. "Cholesterol Measurements: Quality Assurance and Medical Usefulness Interrelationships." *Archives of Pathological Laboratory Medicine* 112 (1988): 387-91.

Page, Irvine H., et al. "Hourly Variations in Serum Cholesterol." *Journal of Atherosclerosis* 2 (1962): 181-85.

Schucker, Beth. "Change in Public Perspective on Cholesterol and Heart Disease: Results from Two National Surveys." *JAMA* 258 (1987): 3527-31.

REFERENCES

Chapter 8

Castelli, William P., et al. "A Population at Risk." *American Journal of Medicine* 80 (1986): supp. 2, 23-32.

Hegsted, D.M., et al. "Quantitative Effects of Dietary Fat on Serum Cholesterol in Man." *American Journal of Clinical Nutrition* 17 (1965): 281-95.

National Heart, Lung, and Blood Institute, U.S. Department of Health and Human Services. *Eating to Lower Your Blood Cholesterol.* NIH Publication No. 87-2920, 1987.

Pennington, Jean A.T., et al. *Bowes & Church's Food Values of Portions Commonly Used* (14th ed.). Philadelphia: Lippincott, 1985.

Chapter 9

Abraham, Zara D., et al. "Three-Week Psyllium-Husk Supplementation: Effect on Plasma Cholesterol Concentrations, Fecal Steroid Excretion, and Carbohydrate Absorption in Men." *American Journal of Clinical Nutrition* 47 (1988): 67-74.

Anderson, James W. *Plant Fiber in Foods.* Lexington: HCF Diabetes Research Foundation, 1986.

Anderson, James W., et al. "Cholesterol-Lowering Effects of Psyllium Hydrophilic Mucilloid for Hypercholesterolemic Men." *Archives of Internal Medicine* 148 (1988): 292-96.

———. "Dietary Fiber: Hyperlipidemia, Hypertension, and Coronary Heart Disease." *American Journal of Gastroenterology* 81 (1986): 1907-19.

———. "Dietary Fiber, Lipids, and Atherosclerosis." *American Journal of Cardiology* 60 (1987): 17G-22G.

———. "Hypercholesterolemic Effects of Oat-Bran or Bean Intake for Hyper cholesterolemic Men." *American Journal of Clinical Nutrition* 40 (1984): 1146-55.

———. "Hypolipidemic Effects of High-Carbohydrate, High-Fiber Diets." *Metabolism* 29 (1980): 551-58.

Burkitt, Denis P., et al. "Effects of Dietary Fibre on Stools and Transit Times, and Its Role in the Causation of Disease." *Lancet* 2 (1972): 1408-11.

Gold, Kurt V., et al. "Oat Bran as a Cholesterol-Reducing Dietary Adjunct in a Young, Healthy Population." *Western Journal of Medicine* 148 (1988): 299-302.

Jenkins, David J.A., et al. "Leguminous Seeds in the Dietary Management of Hyperlipidemia." *American Journal of Clinical Nutrition* 38 (1983): 567-73.

Kirby, Robert W., et al. "Oat-Bran Intake Selectively Lowers Serum Low-Density Lipoprotein Cholesterol Concentrations." *American Journal of Clinical Nutrition* 34 (1981): 824-29.

Sprecher, Dennis L., et al. "Efficacy of Psyllium in Reducing Serum Cholesterol Levels in Hypercholesterolemic Patients on High-or Low-Fat Diets." *Annals of Internal Medicine* 119 (1993): 545-54.

Chapter 10

Barrett-Connor, Elizabeth, et al. "A Community Study of Alcohol and Other Factors Associated with the Distribution of High-Density Lipoprotein Cholesterol in Older vs. Younger Men." *American Journal of Epidemiology* 115 (1982): 888-93.

Blackwelder, William C., et al. "Alcohol and Mortality: The Honolulu Heart Study." *American Journal of Medicine* 68 (1980): 164-69.

Brenn, Tormod. "The Tromso Heart Study: Alcoholic Beverages and Coronary Risk Factors." *Journal of Epidemiology and Community Health* 40 (1986): 249-56.

Criqui, Michael H. "Cigarette Smoking and Plasma High-Density Lipoprotein Cholesterol." *Circulation* 62 (1980): 70-76.

Enger, Sven, et al. "High-Density Lipoproteins (HDL) and Physical Activity: The Influence of Physical Exercise, Age, and Smoking on HDL-Cholesterol and the HDL/Total Cholesterol Ratio." *Scandinavian Journal of Clinical and Laboratory Investigation* 37 (1977): 251-55.

Ernst, Nancy, et al. "The Association of Plasma High-Density Lipoprotein Cholesterol with Dietary Intake and Alcohol Consumption: The Lipid Research Clinics Program Prevalence Study." *Circulation* 62 (1980): supp. 4, 41-52.

Fortmann, Stephen P., et al. "Changes in Plasma High Density Lipoprotein Cholesterol After Changes in Cigarette Use." *American Journal of Epidemiology* 124 (1986): 706-10.

Gordon, David J., et al. "Seasonal Cholesterol Cycles: The Lipid Research Clinics Coronary Primary Prevention Trial Placebo Group." *Circulation* 76 (1987): 1224-31.

Hartung, G. Harley. "Effects of Marathon Running, Jogging, and Diet on Coronary Risk Factors in Middle-Aged Men." *Preventive Medicine* 10 (1981): 316-23.

Haskell, William L. "Strenuous Physical Activity, Treadmill Exercise Test Performance, and Plasma High-Density Lipoprotein Cholesterol." *Circulation* 62 (1980): supp. 4, 53-60.

REFERENCES

Herbert, Peter N., et al. "High-Density Lipoprotein Metabolism in Runners and Sedentary Men." *JAMA* 252 (1984): 1034-37.

Hurt, Richard D., et al. "Plasma Lipids and Apolipoprotein A-I and A-II Levels in Alcoholic Patients." *American Journal of Clinical Nutrition* 43 (1986): 521-29.

Leon, Arthur S., et al. "Leisure-Time Physical Activity Levels and Risk of Coronary Heart Disease and Death: The Multiple Risk Factor Intervention Trial." *JAMA* 258 (1987): 2388-95.

Mattson, F.H., et al. "Effect of Dietary Cholesterol on Serum Cholesterol in Man." *American Journal of Clinical Nutrition* 25 (1972): 589-94.

Phillipson, Beverley E. "Effects of Walking upon Plasma Lipids in Hyperlipidemic Patients." *Alabama Medicine* 53 (November 1983): 15-18.

Renaud, S., et al. "Wine, Alcohol, Platelets, and the French Paradox for Coronary Heart Disease." *Lancet* 339 (1992): 1523-26.

Rippey, Robert M. "Overview: Seasonal Variations in Cholesterol." *Preventive Medicine* 10 (1981): 655-59.

Superko, H.R., et al. "The Role of Exercise Training in the Therapy of Hyperlipoproteinemia." *Cardiology Clinics* 5 (1987): 285-310.

Thompson, Paul D., et al. "Exercise, Diet, or Physical Characteristics as Determinants of HDL Levels in Endurance Athletes." *Atherosclerosis* 46 (1983): 333-39.

Wilson, Peter W.F., et al. "Factors Associated with Lipoprotein Cholesterol Levels: The Framingham Study." *Arteriosclerosis* 3 (1983): 273-81.

Wood, Peter D., et al. "Changes in Plasma Lipids and Lipoproteins in Overweight Men During Weight Loss Through Dieting as Compared with Exercise." *New England Journal of Medicine* 319 (1988): 1173-79.

———. "The Effects on Plasma Lipoproteins of a Prudent Weight-Reducing Diet, with or without Exercise, in Overweight Men and Women." *New England Journal of Medicine* 325 (1991): 461-68.

Yano, Katsuhiko, et al. "Coffee, Alcohol, and Risk of Coronary Heart Disease Among Japanese Men Living in Hawaii." *New England Journal of Medicine* 297 (9177): 405-409.

Chapter 11

Forde, Olav H., et al. "The Tromso Heart Study: Coffee Consumption and Serum Lipid Concentrations in Men with Hypercholesterolemia: A Randomised Intervention Study." *British Medical Journal* 290 (1985): 893-95.

Harris, William S. "Effects of a Low Saturated Fat, Low Cholesterol Fish Oil Supplement in Hypertriglyceridemic Patients." *Annals of Internal Medicine* 109 (1988): 465-70.

Jain, Adesh K., et al. "Can Garlic Reduce Levels of Serum Lipids? A Controlled Clinical Study." *American Journal of Medicine* 94 (1993): 632-35.

Kromhout, Daan. "The Inverse Relation Between Fish Consumption and 20-Year Mortality from Coronary Heart Disease." *New England Journal of Medicine* 312 (1985): 1205-1209.

Leaf, Alexander, et al. "Cardiovascular Effects on n-3 Fatty Acids." *New England Journal of Medicine* 318 (1988): 549-56.

Phillipson, Beverley E., et al. "Reduction of Plasma Lipids, Lipoproteins, and Apoproteins by Dietary Fish Oils in Patients with Hypertriglyceridemia." *New England Journal of Medicine* 312 (1985): 1210-16.

Rimm, Eric B., et al. "Vitamin E Consumption and the Risk of Coronary Heart Disease in Men." *New England Journal of Medicine* 328 (1993): 1450-56.

Sacks, Frank M., et al. "Effects of a Low-Fat Diet on Plasma Lipoprotein Levels." *Archives of Internal Medicine* 146 (1986): 1573-77.

Stampfer, Meir J., et al. "Vitamin E Consumption and the Risk of Coronary Disease in Women." *New England Journal of Medicine* 328 (1993): 1444-49.

Thelle, Dag S., et al. "The Tromso Heart Study: Does Coffee Raise Serum Cholesterol?" *New England Journal of Medicine* 308 (1983): 1454-57.

Warshafsky, Stephen, et al. "Effect of Garlic on Total Serum Cholesterol." *Annals of Internal Medicine* 119 (1993): 599-605.

Chapter 13

Blankenhorn, David H., et al. "Beneficial Effects of Combined Colestipol-Niacin Therapy on Coronary Atherosclerosis and Coronary Venous Bypass Grafts." *JAMA* 257 (1987): 3233-40.

Canner, Paul L., et al. "Fifteen-Year Mortality in Coronary Drug Project Patients: Long-Term Benefits with Niacin." *Journal of the American College of Cardiology* 8 (1986): 1245-55.

Clementz, Gregory L., et al. "Nicotinic Acid-Induced Fulminant Hepatic Failure." *Journal of Clinical Gastroenterology* 9 (1987): 582-84.

Committee of Principal Investigators, WHO Clofibrate Trial. "A Cooperative Trial in the Primary Prevention of Ischemic Heart Disease Using Clofibrate." *British Heart Journal* 40 (1978): 1069-1118.

Coronary Drug Project Research Group. "Clofibrate and Niacin in Coronary Heart Disease." *JAMA* 231 (1975): 360-81.

REFERENCES

Havel, Richard J., et al. "Lovastatin (Mevinolin) in the Treatment of Heterozygous Familial Hypercholesterolemia." *Annals of Internal Medicine* 107 (1987): 609-15.

Hunninghake, Donald B., et al. "The Efficacy of Intensive Dietary Therapy Alone or Combined with Lovastatin in Outpatients with Hypercholesterolemia." *New England Journal of Medicine* 328 (1993): 1213-19.

Illingworth, D. Roger. "Lipid-Lowering Drugs: An Overview of Indications and Optimum Therapeutic Use." *Drugs* 33 (1987): 259-79.

Lipid Research Clinics Program. "The Lipid Research Clinics Coronary Primary Prevention Trial Results." *JAMA* 251 (1984): 351-74.

Lovastatin Study Group II. "Therapeutic Response to Lovastatin (Mevinolin) in Nonfamilial Hypercholesterolemia: A Multicenter Study." *JAMA* 256 (1986): 2829-34.

Malloy, Mary J., et al. "Complementarity of Colestipol, Niacin, and Lovastatin in Treatment of Severe Familial Hypercholesterolemia." *Annals of Internal Medicine* 107 (1987): 616-23.

Manninen, Vesa, et al. "Lipid Alterations and Decline in the Incidence of Coronary Heart Disease in the Helsinki Heart Study." *JAMA* 260 (1988): 641-51.

Multiple Risk Factor Intervention Trial Research Group. "Multiple Risk Factor Intervention Trial, Risk Factor Changes, and Mortality Results." *JAMA* 248 (1982): 1465-77.

Nessim, Sharon A., et al. "Combined Therapy of Niacin, Colestipol, and Fat-Controlled Diet in Men with Coronary Bypass." *Atherosclerosis* 3 (1983): 568-73.

Oster, Gerry, et al. "Cost-Effectiveness of Antihyperlipidemic Therapy in the Prevention of Coronary Heart Disease." *JAMA* 258 (1987): 2381-87.

"Report of the National Cholesterol Education Expert Panel on Detection, Evaluation, and Treatment of High Blood Cholesterol in Adults." *Archives of Internal Medicine* 148 (1988): 36-69.

Roberts, Leslie. "Study Bolsters Case Against Cholesterol." *Science* 237 (1987): 28-29.

Tikkanen, Matti J., et al. "Current Pharmacologic Treatment of Elevated Serum Cholesterol." *Circulation* 76 (1987): 529-33.

INDEX

About the Authors

Dr. Art Ulene has been known to television viewers over the past two decades through his medical reports on the NBC "Today Show" and the ABC "HOME Show." Additionally, he is the author of numerous books and the producer of several video and audio programs. He lives in Los Angeles.

Dr. Ulene's co-author is his daughter, Dr. Val Ulene, also a medical doctor. In addition to the medical degree which she received from Columbia University, Dr. Val Ulene holds a master's degree in public health. She lives in New York City.

Count Out Cholesterol is the second book in a series of health books currently being written by the Ulenes.

OTHER BOOKS BY DR. ART ULENE AND DR. VAL ULENE:

Count Out Cholesterol Cookbook............................$14.95
> A companion guide to *Count Out Cholesterol*, this
> book shows you how to bring your cholesterol
> levels down with the help of 250 gourmet
> recipes.

How to Cut Your Medical Bills..............................$11.95
> Dr. Art Ulene and Dr. Val Ulene investigate how
> the best hospitals, doctors and treatments are
> often the least expensive. Along the way they
> explore how to save on everything from eye-
> glasses and x-rays to health insurance and heart
> surgery.

The Vitamin Strategy..$11.95
> A game plan for good health, this book helps
> readers design a vitamin and mineral program
> tailored to their individual needs.

Discovery Play...$9.95
> By Dr. Art Ulene and Dr. Steven Shelov, this book
> guides readers through the first eighteen months
> of parenting with a special emphasis on nurtur-
> ing self-esteem.

*To order these or other Ulysses Press books call 800-377-
2542 or write to Ulysses Press P.O. Box 3440, Berkeley,
CA 94703-3440. **All retail orders are shipped free of
charge.** California residents must include sales tax. Allow
two to three weeks for delivery.*